Caregiver's Reprieve

Caregiver's Reprieve

A Guide to Emotional Survival When You're Caring for Someone You Love

Avrene L. Brandt, Ph.D.

THE WORKING CAREGIVER SERIES

Impact Publishers®
SAN LUIS OBISPO, CALIFORNIA

Impact Publishers and colophon are registered trademarks of Impact Publishers, Inc.

ATTENTION ORGANIZATIONS AND CORPORATIONS:
This book is available at quantity discounts on bulk purchases for educational, business, or sales promotional use. For further information, please contact Impact Publishers, P.O. Box 910, San Luis Obispo, California 93406-0910 (Phone: 1-800-246-7228).

Library of Congress Cataloging-in-Publication Data

Brandt, Avrene L.-
    Caregiver's reprieve : a guide to emotional survival when you're caring for someone you love / Avrene L. Brandt.
        p.   cm. ---- (The working caregiver series)
    Includes bibliographical references and index.
    ISBN 1-886230-06-4 (alk. paper)
    1. Chronically ill----Home care----Psychological aspects.
    2. Caregivers. 3. Aged----Home care----Psychological aspects.
    I. Title.   II. Series.
RC108.B7   1997
362.1'01'9----dc21   97-28261
                                                                CIP

Publisher's Note
This publication is designed to provide accurate and authoritative information in regard to the subject matter covered. It is sold with the understanding that the publisher is not engaged in rendering psychological, medical, or other professional services. If expert assistance or counseling is needed, the services of a competent professional should be sought.

Printed in the United States of America on acid-free paper
Cover design by Sharon Schnare, San Luis Obispo, California

Published by **Impact 🐌 Publishers**®
POST OFFICE BOX 910
SAN LUIS OBISPO, CALIFORNIA 93406-0910

To my father, who spoke to me with his eyes.

CONTENTS

PREFACE

Between the verdict and the sentence, between the overture and the finale, is the reprieve. A reprieve is not a pardon. A reprieve does not mean that you are home free. A reprieve is a temporary stay that grants time.

And in that time, when it begins to feel as though it will never be the same, and the roles change and the dreams change and the future changes, and one of you becomes responsible for getting both of you through it, then you become the caregiver.

ACKNOWLEDGEMENTS

I wish to thank my family for their enthusiasm and support in this venture.

I wish to express my appreciation to those professionals who assisted me, especially Dr. Raymond H. Coll for his input and Dr. and Mrs. Morrie Kricun for confirming the merit of *Caregiver's Reprieve*.

I would also like to acknowledge the caregivers I have met through the Greater Philadelphia chapter of the Alzheimer's Association, in my practice, and especially my mother, for making me aware of the importance of writing this book.

Finally, I am grateful to my friends who cared and were there for me in my own time of loss.

INTRODUCTION

M r. C, a neatly groomed, fiftyish man, arrived for his first session. He entered my office and sat down in the farther of the two single patient chairs. His shoulders turned in toward his body, and he barely met my glance. He had been referred by the local Adult Protective Services for suspected physical abuse of his elderly Alzheimer's-impaired mother. It was suspected that, on several occasions, in the course of his caring for her, he had mistreated her. During his treatment, however, he only acknowledged one episode in which he had lost control. His shame was intense. He had never thought of himself as an angry or hurtful person.

Mrs. L. was an attractive 37-year-old woman who held her hands together in an effort to control her fidgeting. She explained that although she was doing much better, she continued to have moments of extreme anxiety during which she had trouble keeping her hands still. Her therapy sessions were one component of her outpatient treatment — she had recently been released from a 30-day alcohol rehabilitation program. Although Mrs. L. did not report a history of alcohol addiction, both her paternal grandfather and one brother had drinking problems. Her problem with alcohol had begun eleven months into her role of caregiver for her husband, who was stricken with a rapidly progressing case of multiple sclerosis. She described her exhaustion from the daily stresses of caregiving, her lack of support, and her fear of eventual loss. These were so overwhelming that the relief associated with a bottle of brandy became an irresistible call.

Current estimates suggest that there are seven million *caregivers* in the United States ---- individuals who are primarily responsible for the health, maintenance and care of an aged or chronically ill loved one. With ever increasing medical advances contributing to extended longevity, it is estimated that in the next thirty years, the population of elderly will double. Furthermore, the highest increase will be in the more frail age bracket ---- 75 years and older.

Most of today's elderly are not in nursing homes. In fact, 70-80% of the elderly are cared for by their families. For caregivers, that can mean a commitment of between ten and twenty years.

The challenge of caregiving has recently received considerable attention. This is largely due to a growing awareness of the impact that cognitive impairments, such as those associated with Alzheimer's Disease, have on families. There is now a considerable body of literature and an increase in attention to the stresses and consequences of caring for a chronically ill loved one. Through the efforts of many local and national organizations, as well as individual chronicles, caregivers have a greatly improved network of support and information. Excellent resources exist to help families with the daily routine of caregiving, as well as special issues such as medical, legal and long term planning. Numerous publications and support systems have appeared which deal with the practical issues of caregiving. Many caregivers' journals have been published in books. To a lesser degree, some research and a few publications have dealt with the emotional aspects of caregiving.

In contrast to the increase in practical information and personal stories, there is still a relative scarcity of books which address the *emotional stress* of caregiving. As a consultant and lecturer for the Alzheimer's Association, as well as in my role as a support group facilitator, I have received repeated feedback from group members attesting to their need for information to help them deal with their emotional reactions, not only to the traumatic, but also to the daily aspects of caregiving.

The intent of *Caregiver's Reprieve*, therefore, is to provide information about the emotional travails caregivers encounter, to reassure them of the normality of their feelings, and to aid in the resolution of their feelings.

In this book you will meet four caregiver families. I have endeavored to create emotionally real caregivers, and they are, in fact, a composite of many individuals I have met in my clinical practice. Perhaps you will find yourself in their words and perhaps their renewal will give you comfort.

The book is organized into three general sections. It begins, as caregivers do, with a diagnosis or crisis, which brings a change to life as previously known. Subsequently, as happens with the caregiver, there is the preparation and assembling of information. The first chapters of the book, therefore, provide general information and an overview of caregiving. The book then concentrates on the interplay between altered life expectations, coping styles and emotional responses. This interplay is clarified through the four caregivers who portray the emotions described.

Finally, the book seeks to move you (the caregiver) beyond catastrophe to resolution ---- a coming to terms with tragedy and loss. It encourages re-examination of personal philosophies and commitment to life beyond caregiving.

Appendix chapters on brain functions and medical information are included as a basic framework for readers who wish to know more about symptomatology and treatment. These sections are meant to be used as a basic reference and are not intended to provide comprehensive neurological information.

It is my hope that this book will help you gain strength, understanding, self-acceptance, and the reprieve which will enable you to reinvest in life.

1

THE CAREGIVERS

Becca

April 1988. Warm April evening. Scent of spring in the air. Spirits stretching forward to uncoil and unwrap in May colors...

The ominous jolt of the telephone in the night. Hardly awake, Becca reached for the phone and glanced at the clock: 11:20.

"Mrs. Haney? Is this the Haney residence?"

"Yes, this is Mrs. Haney."

"Mrs. Haney, this is Dr. Phelp at Richfield Hospital. We have your son, Brian, here. He's been brought into the hospital. There's been an accident. He's being treated in the Emergency Room. Can you come now?"

"Yes, yes! Is he all right?" *(Fear, the alarm of imminent danger, the panic associated with uncertainty. Fear is a siren for the caregiver.)*

"Your son appears to have sustained some serious injuries. You can come directly to the Emergency Room."

"Tom." Becca turned to her husband, now roused by the edge in her voice. "It's Brian." Her words choking her, felt like the gasp of a struggling swimmer. "He's in the hospital. An accident."

Often in the times that followed she would try to remember that first moment of alarm. A hazy memory except for the vague sense of being in the car, until her first glimpse of Brian between the white cotton coats working over him in the Emergency Room.

Could she say she was altogether unprepared for this? No. Of her three children, Brian had never been easy. Becca, with her expectations and her need for order, was continually reminded that Brian had a mind of his own. As a small child he had been moved by the impulse of the moment. In grade school he had a "come whatever" attitude, and in adolescence he developed a "free spirit" outlook Becca did not understand.

Brian, now nineteen, had the air of someone just entering adolescence, untamed. His dark, unshaped hair hung below his ears, often accented by untended facial stubble.

She remembered their recent encounter, a week earlier. Brian had said he expected that his low grades would result in his being asked to leave college at the end of the second semester.

"Hey, Mom," he had said. "Look, you know I never liked this school stuff. Randy is Mr. College."

Becca remembered feeling frustrated as she watched him. He shifted his feet about, not meeting her glance, probably not hearing what she was saying. She had not connected with him and this was likely to be another one of their archaic, racquetball battles.

Yet, there in his eyes, she caught a softening playing behind the familiar cobalt blue, as if he, too, were tired of sparring. She took a breath. "Won't you just try school for one more year? Maybe you'll find something you like."

"Mom, I know..." he began, but then stopped. His body eased. "O.K., I'll go to Community College for a year, but you've got to let me have the bike, so I can take it cross-country with Sarah this summer."

The bike. The Yamaha that she and Tom had co-signed for. The bike that he had ridden this April evening, now damaged and out of commission, like her son.

Becca sat with Tom in the room where the paramedic had led them. She was able to see the doctors and nurses working around Brian. Her body was tense with the anxiety of not knowing, except for the brief moment when one of the doctors had come out and explained the severity of Brian's injuries. He had ended with,

"He's alive. We have that," and then quickly excused himself, promising to return as soon as possible. Alive ---- the first reprieve.

Tom Haney, age 52, and Rebecca Haney (née Gruber), age 49, married 27 years. Three children: Randy, 25; Meredith, 23; Brian, 19. Tom, Senior Research Director at Fielding Labs. Rebecca, Manager, Accounts Receivable at Sloan's Department Store.

Rebecca Gruber: Class of '57, Cedarcrest High School. Class Treasurer, yearbook staff member, French Achievement Award recipient, and manager of Girls Softball team. Married Tom Haney in 1963 after finishing junior college. (Tom: agreeable, easygoing, hard working, and content to let Becca make the decisions).

Becca Haney: Careful, orderly, scheduled, organized. Becca's credo: She is willing to do whatever is needed to achieve her goal. She knows that if she is careful and organized, everything will work out.

Sitting in the waiting room, Becca noticed that she was grateful for Tom's silence beside her, allowing her to think. She was acutely aware of the unbearable tension of not knowing details and not being able to do anything. She felt herself holding back from pressing the emergency room physicians, fearful that if she were not right there watching, Brian might die before she could direct them to save him ---- or save him herself. Her mind strayed back to a July day when the children were young.

The boys had found a fledgling bird in the driveway. They told her that for several mornings they had heard the bird chirping in the driveway. Becca had gone out and found the small brownish bird, its feathers puffed up, its eyes small slits, and its beak open, exhausted from being in the sun.

They decided to try to save the bird. It took some time to catch it. Repeatedly, the small bird gathered its strength to flutter away on the ground, its instincts moving it to frenzy.

Finally they caught the bird and fashioned a nest-like structure in a box with slats on the side. The little bird, still unable to fly, took worms and bread and water from them. It chirped incessantly that first day, frequently opening its mouth so wide for food that the pink and orange of its mouth eclipsed the rest of its body.

Becca called the Wildlife Center to find out what to do about the bird. A baby robin, it was. The Wildlife people advised that if the bird's mother had been feeding it on the ground, as was likely, the bird should be let go.

"Return it to a safe place as soon as possible, and watch to see if the mother bird feeds it. Wait a day," they advised because rain was in the forecast.

The next morning Becca went to check the bird. The box was quiet. She lifted the lid and looked inside. There sat the little bird, perfectly dead, facing ahead, as if, in a brief moment, it had simply died. Becca noticed that on the lid of the box were two paw prints; probably a dog or raccoon had tried to get in. Perhaps the fledgling had died of fright.

Randy and Brian buried the bird in the back, near the turtle that had been hit on the road.

Coming back to the house, Becca heard the noise. Loud, throaty, sharp chirping. There, perched at the very edge of a nearby maple branch, dangled a red-breasted robin, positioned where it could see the entire event. Persistently calling as Becca passed, "Why didn't you let me take care of my own?" Other hands had tended her baby, and now the fledgling was dead. Becca stopped, faced the bird, and lowered her head in acknowledgment. The bird had paused, caught in Becca's contrition, and then flew away.

Now Becca looked toward the room where the staff worked on Brian: tubes in his arms, a monitor attached to his chest, and a pump rhythmically pushing air into his lungs. She felt the tightness in her throat.

Fred

June 1987. Heads look up to the clink of a fork against fine stemware as glasses are lifted. A slightly overweight, balding man in a dark blue suit addresses the gathering.

"Ladies and gentlemen, a toast to the man of the evening, Fred Krasner, retiring after 35 years, looking forward to more time with Ruth, his beautiful wife of 37 years, and to his much-loved game of golf.

"Fred joined Harwell Corporation when we were a new company. He was always a team player and eventually a member of the executive circle. He is known for his calm under pressure and his ability to get things to work and come together. As Fred leaves his position as Senior Vice President, we offer this toast from his friends and co-workers. To Fred and Ruth. Salute!"

October 1927. Saturday mornings. Fred's mother would go off with his sister, Carla. Fred, at age five, accompanied his father to W. & H. Paper Company where Mr. Krasner, the mill foreman, did the Saturday morning check on operations.

Fred observed his father nod here and comment there, in passing. Occasionally, his father bent down to whisper to Fred and repeat what he had said: Joseph, the stocky, curly haired man in the blue shirt got a warning about his tendency to come in late; Mike, the new man on the press, too often confused, was likely to be moved. Pete, dependable and an old timer, got a pat on the shoulder.

Fred watched as his father "positioned" them and then thought about how he liked to move his Army figures on his plastic battlefield at home. He imagined his own crew, saw himself tall like his father, directing, placing, gently rotating the figures, a kind sergeant in the field.

March 1941. In his sophomore year at Penn State, Fred had a roommate, Lew. A tall, well-built, Main Line Philadelphian, Lew was self-indulgent and quick to give vent to his anger when frustrated. Fred and Lew found themselves together in Statistics II with Professor Cready — a constricted, methodical, sixtyish teacher with a disdain for pleasure, pretense, and that which could not be precisely defined. Lew, impulsive and self-absorbed, did not stand in good stead with Professor Cready, and, by association, neither did Fred.

Exams were graded both for understanding of the statistical concepts and for correctness of the answer, but there was no consistency as to how Cready would weigh the factors on any given exam. March midterm grades were a disappointment. Lew came up with a D, Fred a C-. No partial credit was given on the proofs. Lew was quick to feel cheated and compared his answers with classmates who appeared to have gotten partial credit. Fred saw the discrepancy, but opted to accept that he had not studied enough. Lew confronted Cready, his football frame hovering over the Professor, as he demanded a review of his paper. But Cready had the ball. Fred swallowed his own frustration. What was the point? He didn't see himself making a fuss. Lew was not going to win. You can't always blitz the quarterback. That was not how Dad played in the field.

February 1988. Ruth was preening again. Making sure she looked just right. At 61 years of age, she still took pride in being an attractive woman; dark hazel eyes, curly graying hair, and skin as smooth as a young woman's. Fred was pleased to be seen with her.

Lately, she took longer to get ready, but Fred didn't mind. He had time, now that he was retired. The years of working hard were worth it. Now he and Ruth could enjoy these years comfortably.

"Ruth, Ruth, what's the hold up?" He walked into the bedroom.

Ruth was sitting on the bed, struggling with her clothes, trying to put a mauve, long-sleeved blouse over her bulky white sweater.

"Ruthie, the blouse goes underneath. Here, let me help you." *What was she doing?*

"Of course, I'm so foolish. I couldn't get it right. What's the matter with me? I must have gotten tangled up in the sleeve."

November 1988. Fred listened to the neurologist as he explained the findings.

"How have you been? Sit down please. Well... all the tests are completed and we have been able to eliminate most of the disorders which result in the symptoms Ruth is showing. We know that it isn't a thyroid disorder or a brain tumor or a problem with metabolism or depression. What we are left with is a memory disorder that is age-related, and that, unfortunately, does not improve with time."

Dr. Mellman waited for questions. Ruth sat quietly, but Fred wanted to know what they could expect. Dr. Mellman briefly noted some of the difficulties that might develop and then encouraged Fred to call if he had further questions.

It was November, and Fred noticed advertisements on television announcing that it was National Alzheimer's Month. He called Dr. Mellman's office.

"Is it like Alzheimer's?" he asked the doctor.

"Yes, the picture is consistent with Alzheimer's, but there is no conclusive test for Alzheimer's at this time."

Dr. Mellman then explained more about Alzheimer's for Fred, closing with, "Remember, please call me if you notice unusual behaviors or changes that concern you."

November 15, 1988. Fred came home after a short round of golf. The weather was turning brisk and he did not like leaving Ruth alone for long periods of time now. He opened the refrigerator door and reached for the orange juice. Sardines! The smell of sardines. A half empty tin of sardines near the front of the second shelf. Perplexed, he instinctively looked on the floor. In a little white bowl, like the one they used to have for Miriam, Ruth's cat, was the other half of the tin of sardines. But Miriam had been dead for seven years.

Fred wondered if he should call Dr. Mellman, but decided against it.

Nora

March, 1988. When the shadow in Glenn's stomach was diagnosed as a malignancy, Nora was terrified. The verdict stripped away the security she had known in being married to Glenn and left her in a state of panic.

Seven years earlier, at age 27, Nora had married Glenn Tolbert, eight years her senior. She had met him shortly after the termination of her affair with a professor she had met in her junior year at college. The professor had finally declared that their relationship was static and that he could not envision himself married to the beautiful, but guileless, Nora.

Nora, in her lonely despair, then met recently divorced Glenn, whose ex-wife had not wanted children. Glenn was taken by the neediness and naivete of the dark-haired, waifish Nora. Their marriage was compatible, without much excitement.

Glenn was protective, steadfast, and practical. "You need and I will provide."

Nora was compliant. "You say how and I will listen."

Glenn: "You wait and I will return."

Nora: "Keep me warm and I will love you forever."

May 12, 1959. Nora is six today. She is dressed in a white ruffled dress with red polka dots that brings out the darkness of her eyes. Her chestnut hair, held back with a red barrette, streams down her back. The red ribbon around her hat matches the polka dots of her dress, and Nora is a doll today. Nora is Daddy's girl, her hand tucked in his, as he parades his Nora doll. She is secure, knowing that he will always take care of her.

June 1973. Nora had attended a liberal arts college in the North. Daddy's intent had been to provide her with an opportunity to acquire some sophistication. Nora had little idea of why she was in college or what she wanted to study, but she followed her father's direction.

Nora was quickly overwhelmed by the pace of college and was relieved to be absorbed by one of the prestigious sororities. There she partied and drank a little. Her selection of English as a major was convenient, but not inspired, until her junior year. It was at that point that Richard, her Comparative Literature professor, took a protective interest in her. Subsequently, under his tutelage, she buckled down and made an acceptable foray into her studies.

Upon graduation, she and Richard began a three-year affair. Richard was insightful and decisive. Nora was receptive, accommodating and comfortable.

April 1988. Now, for the first time, Nora sat in the small hospital chapel, while above, the surgeons worked to excise the potential spoiler of her dreams.

"Are you afraid?" she had asked Glenn, the words touching her own fear, hoping that if he did not feel fear, then there was really nothing to be afraid of.

Woody

February 1968. "Woody!"

"*Hey, Jude, don't make it bad. Take a sad song and make it better...*"

"Woody!"

"*Remember to let her under your skin, then you can start...*"

He stalled, not wanting to answer. Turned off the radio. "Ya, Mam," and started toward the kitchen before she could call again. Her call grated him. Always something he had done wrong or something she'd be needing him to do, nowadays that she had spells of feeling tired and weak ---- "Peaked," she said.

This was not the Mam who raised them. Mam had been tireless, undaunted, and in charge ---- even before she and Pop split when Woody was eight.

Mam had come from Ireland with her family, post WWII. Her father came over first with his brother and saved up till he could bring the family over. Mam (Kathleen) was 18 then. The family was poor, but Kathleen was determined not to feel humble, like a foreigner. She dreamed American dreams.

Mam fell in love with Patrick Leary, and they married when she was 21. Then there was Woody, then Megan, then Patrick's drinking, and then she knew that dreams don't necessarily cross with reality.

Woody looked at her now as he came into the kitchen. Her face ---- somewhat square and hard, framed with dark red hair ---- was still young. She was tired though, like an old woman, although she was just 38 years old. In the past year or so she seemed to have less energy but more irritation. He had always thought of her as irritable and critical ---- even when he and Megan were young ---- telling him he'd never come up to much, saying he'd be like his father, the "bummer." Patrick, of course, had the good fortune to have been liberated from her and had hardly ever made contact with them in years.

Now he bristled at the sound of her calling his name, remembering how she could always make him feel: inadequate, powerless, chattled. But he was used to heeding her, especially of late, since she seemed to need him more, now that she had spells of feeling poorly.

Woody thought back...

Winter 1961. "Woody! Get ye' clothes. Put 'em in th' bags and help Megan with hers. We're leavin', and this time for good."

She'd said that before and they'd gone and come back. Why didn't they just keep the stuff in them ugly brown bags?

This time, though, they didn't go to Grandma Hogan's. This time they had a place of their own, and this time they never went back. Home was a small, gray apartment where Pop was not welcome and hardly ever came to see them.

Mam, of course, grousin' about Pop's wasting the support money on the drink. Grousin' and spoutin' and maybe rightly so, but Woody didn't want to hear it. It rubbed a nerve that was already tender.

They all work hard to keep things up. Mam complains a lot. Megan and he silently endure. Megan is a quiet, compliant girl with fear on her face. Woody sometimes is disgusted by her fear and sometimes feels sorry for her. Mostly he feels resentment for Mam. He finds an escape because he is a good athlete and Mam is proud of that. He plays seasonal sports on the school teams and escapes for practice and games. He uses it to get away from her call. When she complains about his absence, he says, "The team needs me." Later he tells her about his part in the wins and she nods (her closest concession to his worth), but she had quickly followed with, "And now if only we could see ye' grades come up to that."

Why had it always ended with him feeling angry?

1969. Well, so now they said there was a reason why she'd become so tired and irritable. Mam was diagnosed with multiple sclerosis.

He thinks, *That explains the last five years, but what about the other twelve years that he's known her?* Now what will happen to his plan to leave next year when he turns 18, now that she'll be needing him?

Mrs. Miller, two doors down, is affiliated with God and talks to Woody about his being strong for Mam. The glory of helping. She encourages him to look to the future with hope. She talks to him about Sal DiPietro — such a good son — who cares for his mother who has Alzheimer's. From her mouth it sounds like a holy crusade, a glorious challenge, a path to the Kingdom of Heaven. What does she know? Easy for her to say. Did Sal's mother criticize everything he did? Was she never satisfied? Did Sal's mother expect him to be at her beck and call? Did yours, Mrs. Miller?

2

CAREGIVING: AN OVERVIEW

I t is probably not a subject that would have caught your attention. If mentioned, perhaps it would have aroused mild to moderate sympathy ---- similar, perhaps, to the feelings for the abandoned, disabled children in Romania or for the hardship of the Indians in New Delhi. But now you are the caregiver, and now you *must* pay attention.

Caregiving permeates all aspects of life ---- the practical, the emotional, the physical and the spiritual. The scope of the role affects your plans, dreams, identity and beliefs. Caregiving is treading water twenty-four hours a day, surrounded by currents that exhaust your ability to stay afloat. To be a caregiver is to know that unfair things can happen, that your life with your loved one is all changed about, and that you are challenged.

At the beginning, there is the preparation, which involves collecting information, gathering a team, building a support system which includes family, medical, legal and social service components. Soon it becomes apparent that illnesses that require caregiving often cause significant mental, as well as physical, changes in the loved one. As a result, the nature of the quality of the relationship between the caregiver and the loved one shifts. For the son or daughter of an impaired parent, the parent becomes the child and the child becomes the parent. When the caregiver is the parent of an adult child or adolescent, the parent must accept a responsibility that promises to restrict forever her or his freedom, independence and future plans.

Spouses who become caregivers find that the partnership has changed. Roles, expectations, and the fulfillment of needs are altered. Daily routines are increasingly disrupted, as are work schedules, leisure times, social activities, rest and recreation. Mutual dependency, sharing and intimacy change, diminish, and can be lost if new ways of connecting are not made. The loss of the familiar, the loved, the assumed, precipitates depression. Losses appear to outweigh gains, struggles replace rewards, and the past is envied because the future appears gloomy.

Depression is a normal reaction to loss; however, *clinical depression* ---- feelings of hopelessness, intense sadness, irritability, sleep and/or appetite disturbances ---- may occur and signal that the stress is exceeding the coping ability of the caregiver.

Depression is certainly not the only emotion which exists for the caregiver, however. A host of unwelcome emotions emerge. Fear, frustration, anger, despair, guilt, sadness, anxiety, helplessness, confusion, loneliness, are all common.

It is not a subject that would have caught your attention, and if you speak about it, will you be heard?

3

THE LOSS OF
THE PERSON YOU KNEW

Chronic illness can effect the mental, as well as the physical, state of a loved one. Changes in thinking and personality can also be a direct result of underlying brain dysfunction, and are symptoms of the medical condition termed "dementia."

The derivation of the word dementia comes from the Latin prefix *de,* meaning to lessen or reduce, and the root word *mentis,* which is associated with the mind or mental processes. Dementia refers to a deterioration of mental and/or cognitive abilities. Contrary to popular usage of the word "demented," which has a negative connotation, "dementia" labels a medical condition. To the caregiver, however, it is a sentence which forecasts the depersonalization of a loved one.

The cognitive impairment characteristic of dementia can come on suddenly, as a result of a traumatic brain injury, or slowly, as a consequence of a progressive neurological disorder. If the neurological disorder progresses slowly, the behavior and personality changes of the loved one may be puzzling, but not initially recognized as a disease process. In the elderly, these changes may be attributed to advancing age. Families who do not realize that there is a neurological basis for the changes may think that their loved one is being manipulative or lazy. When their efforts to encourage independence are unsuccessful, they begin to feel frustrated, angry and, subsequently, guilty.

One day though, something happens: the person asks the same question repeatedly, or gets lost or disoriented, or shows a disturbance in thinking ---- perhaps a peculiar use of words ---- or cannot remember what was just said. Then it becomes clear that "something is wrong."

The course of a progressive, neurological illness is downhill, because once destroyed, nerve cells do not regenerate.

Early in the illness, when the patient is still functional and can comprehend and express himself/herself in language, the caregiver maintains a level of optimism. Gradually though, the continued losses ---- of skills, independent functioning, the ability to communicate, and memory ---- rob the patient of the ability to interact and be involved in life in a meaningful way.

As the illness progresses it affects the patient's ability to complete previously learned tasks. Disorientation of time and place disrupt daily schedules. Impairment in planning, organizing and sustaining interest interfere with the performance of more complex projects. In time, even routine tasks, including dressing and maintaining hygiene, become problematic. Confusion about sequencing results in disorganized attempts at dressing. Peculiar eating behaviors may be observed.

> *June 1990.* Fred remembered Ruth at the restaurant on their first date — so proper about what she ordered. He glanced at her now as she reached for the ketchup bottle, opened it and tipped it toward her salad.
>
> Fred watched tensely. "What are you doing?" He gestured to the triangle, of Ruth's hand, the ketchup bottle, and the salad.
>
> Ruth looked up, blank. "What? I... uhhh." A glob of red plopped against the green leaves on her plate.

Along with loss of abilities comes a gradual, increasing dependency on the family for physical and financial assistance. Patients attempt to compensate for their loss of autonomy with clinging or controlling behavior. This is particularly evident in new and complex situations. The caregiver, facing an overwhelming challenge to maintain the status quo, begins to feel inadequate.

Compounding this is the caregiver's fear that the patient's disorientation and diminished ability to think logically will result in something harmful or dangerous. As the patient becomes more dependent, a paradox emerges for the caregiver.

The "dependency paradox" evolves as the caregiver's life increasingly begins to hinge on the dependency of the patient. The caregiver becomes reluctant to leave the loved one and is actually restricted by never-ending needs, schedules and crises. Caregivers who characteristically thought of themselves as independent and in control now experience a loss of control. Life revolves around the patient. When things do not work out as planned, you may begin to feel frustrated and helpless. Caregivers who never felt comfortable making decisions and who preferred depending on others now find the tables are turned. They now have to take charge and inevitably are confronted with self-doubt.

Who is the dependent one and who is independent? Who is controlled and who is in control?

In the declining picture, neither the loss of physical function nor the diminished cognitive ability is as distressing as the changes in your loved one's personality. The face, voice, smile, posture are the same, but the person seems to slip away in bits and pieces, and even, at times, to become someone else. This, too, is at first subtle and inconsistent, so that initially you may be the only one to notice the changes.

In the early stages of disease, the patient maintains a degree of self-awareness and knows that things are not quite right. For the impaired person, this becomes highly anxiety-arousing. Until there is a medical diagnosis, the resulting anxiety, demandingness, and increasing dependency can be confusing for the family. Moreover, as self-esteem and self-confidence deteriorate, the patient exhibits moodiness, fearfulness and withdrawal.

Depression is also a common emotional reaction of the patient with chronic illness. The loss of the ability to function is similar to any loss, whether it be the loss of a loved one, a job, or a dream. There is also scientific research which suggests that changes in brain tissue following disease or trauma can produce depression. The persistence of depression in the loved one is difficult for the caregiver to accept and can intensify feelings of inadequacy and guilt.

Another troublesome set of problems which frequently accompany compromised cognitive functioning are impaired perceptions and reduced judgement in social situations. Patients lose the ability to understand the consequences of their behavior, lack empathy for the needs of others, and then behave in a self-centered or idiosyncratic manner, which, at times, is socially inappropriate. Often, as a result of missing social cues, they become unable to read people's reactions, gestures, and tones of voice. They lose awareness of their own behavior and its effect on others.

As cognitive functioning continues to decline, some patients may display uncontrolled, impulsive and consequently unpredictable behavior. Emotional outbursts, strange table manners, and inappropriate sexual behavior can be manifested. Some patients become very rigid and repetitive in their routines because they cannot deal with new situations. Others become quite anxious, emotionally erratic and clinging, since they feel a loss of control.

Some chronically ill individuals, although cognitively spared, are affected emotionally by the stress of illness. They also may experience anxiety, loss of control, complicated dependency issues and moodiness. In contrast to individuals who become more clingy, some seek emotional distance and try to avoid dependency. They may reject caregiver overtures due to their own anger, fear, frustration and denial about their illness.

If the caregiver and loved one are unable to express their feelings and concerns about the illness, they become at risk for a dysfunctional relationship. Instead of working together in the face of illness, the illness undermines the relationship and puts it in jeopardy.

All of the changes noted in this chapter present the caregiver with a variety of logistical challenges. It is, however, often the caregiver's own unexpected emotional reactions that are the most draining, most conflict-producing, and most in need of reprieve.

If you're confronted with similar challenges and reactions, you may find the information and coping strategies offered in the following chapters helpful.

4

THE CLOTHES WE WEAR

Everyone has a credo, a personal philosophy or attitude toward life which says, "I believe that if I do this and such and conduct my life in this way, then such and such will follow, and things will be the way I want." The construct of the personal credo was thus described by psychologist Ken Moses (1992) in his discourse on loss and grief. The credo shapes your behavior, plans, expectations and relationships. It is the outline into which you fit your life. Like most people, you believe that to the extent that you adhere to the outline, good things will happen to you.

The credo, or personal philosophy, is learned in childhood. Early on, we become aware that there is a big difference between how we'd like the world to be (that is, safe, nurturing and pleasurable), and how the world really is (that being, non-protective, painful and frustrating). In the face of this discrepancy and the resulting feeling of anxiety —— the child adopts a credo which translates roughly thus: "This is the nature of the universe, this is what the world is really like, my beliefs, and this is my place in it. This is how I have to be, or what I have to do in order to avoid pain and gain pleasure" (Moses, 1992).

Your childhood philosophy develops into a personal attitude toward life and is expressed in beliefs and behavior. It guides attachments to people, jobs and goals. You become attached through your hopes, dreams, expectations, plans and wishes.

The credo has further usefulness in that it protects you from the frightening awareness that you are a mortal, vulnerable being. It also provides you with a persona, or mask (Jung, 1923). The persona is *worn*, and it conforms to the requirements of the environment. It is the posture you assume vis-a-vis the world.

What is *worn* can take on several guises. For example, there is the guise of *compliancy*, which says, "If I do everything I should, if only I am good enough and do what is expected, then I will get what I want." The guise of the *player/manipulator* contends, "If I learn how to work the system, if I outsmart it, and if I play it right, then I will get what I want." The guise or credo of the *reactor* asserts, "If I stand up to it, if I stay in there and fight, then I will get what I want."

All credos have the following three basic tenets: One, there is a grand scheme, or higher order, by which life is governed. Two, the grand scheme is logical, and it works. And three, if you adhere to the grand scheme well enough, you will be safe, and good things will happen to you.

The credo can be couched in religious beliefs that sound like this: One, God is all-powerful. Two, God is just and fair. And three, if I am a good person and am righteous and heedful of God, then he will protect me and insure that I am treated with kindness and fairness.

When Things Go Wrong

Typically your personal philosophy serves you well enough and gets you through a good part of your life until something happens: a loss, an unexpected illness, or a catastrophe which jogs your belief system. Then, unexpectedly, your old ways of adapting do not work anymore. You are again unsafe and without answers. Unprotected, and in extreme pain, you are forced to re-examine your philosophy. To survive, you must find an alternative way of coping.

When things go dreadfully wrong, however, most of us initially avoid questioning our basic beliefs. To question might allow that there is unfairness and disorder in the world, and this is disquieting. Abandoning your personal philosophy shakes your foundation and leaves you undefined and vulnerable. Instead, you question yourself or the world. You suppose you were not smart enough, careful enough, attentive enough; the doctor did not know enough, the medics were not fast enough, something was not good enough, and, therefore, it did not work. The world is to blame, and the myth of the credo is briefly preserved in the belief that if you do better or work harder, order will be restored.

In the examining room of a highly regarded breast surgeon, there is a poster on the wall. It shows a doleful-looking white puppy lying down, saying, "I keep mending my ways, Lord, but the stitches keep breaking."

As time and effort do not change the ominous picture, the caregiver gradually begins to accept that things will not get better. The realization sets in that *life does not play by the rules*. The first tenet begins to waver with the thought that the world is not always governed by order ---- the grand scheme has a flaw. The emotions which accompany this are frustration and disbelief.

With appearance of unexpected and unpredictable crises, the second tenet is threatened. The caregiver senses that the world is not a safe place. *Life can be unfair.* Emotionally, this revelation elicits fear and anger.

The last tenet to fall is that we have some control over our mortality, and that by doing good and right we will be safe and nurtured. In actuality, *even if we follow the plan, we may not win.* The emotions associated with the dissolution of this final belief are dread and existential anxiety. We become aware of our vulnerability, limitations and, ultimately, our mortality.

Defending Yourself

To protect yourself while previously held beliefs are dissolving, you may put on another protective layer of "clothing." This supplementary layer is called a *psychological defense system*.

Everyone has defenses ---- psychological mechanisms which protect us from feelings or conflicts that are potentially overwhelming and disruptive to our functioning. Anxiety, guilt, anger, pain, fear and depression are common emotions encountered in the course of caregiving. Psychological defenses, which are learned early in life, reduce the tension and stress associated with feelings and conflicts. Examples of defenses employed to protect against being overwhelmed by these emotions include:

- DENIAL ---- the rejection or blocking from awareness of painful thoughts or feelings. Denial permits a lack of acceptance of reality. That which is not acknowledged does not exist.

  Becca knew that Brian had sustained serious brain injury but she could not acknowledge that he would never be the same.

- ISOLATION ---- the separation of feelings surrounding an idea from the facts, the splitting off of emotions from the thoughts and actions with which they usually occur. If a thought causes too unpleasant a feeling, the feeling is set aside and disconnected from the thought. Thus one can think of something negative without experiencing a negative feeling.

  Becca acknowledged that Brian would always be impaired, but she kept busy and would not allow herself to get depressed about it.

- RATIONALIZATION ---- the justifying, explaining, or making reasonable that which is not reasonable. Rationalization is the substitution of a somewhat plausible explanation for the real one in order to make it more acceptable. It is finding a good reason rather than accepting the actual reason something exists.

  Becca realized that Brian would always be limited in his achievement, but she rationalized that he was never one to have made future plans for himself anyway.

- DISPLACEMENT ---- the transferring of an emotion from an original idea or thing to which it was attached, to another idea, to which it should not be attached. When the original thought is too emotionally charged, the focus of the emotion is changed. Thus the anxiety is transferred to a thought or goal which is not as emotionally arousing.

> Becca was terrified that Brian would not recover, but she focused instead on her concern that the treatment team was not coordinating his program well.

The use of defenses is not a sign of weakness. Defenses are a necessary part of our psychological makeup. Their use begins in childhood, when preferred defenses are developed. Psychological defenses are unconscious mechanisms which come into play when we are in danger of being overwhelmed by stress or emotions. Because they are unconscious mechanisms and we are not typically aware that we are using them, they are not under our control. Therefore they cannot be used selectively. Defenses can make us lose touch with the emotional part of our being, for when we disconnect ourselves from pain in order not to feel, we disconnect ourselves from good feelings, too.

Used in moderation, defenses allow you to continue functioning. Overused, they can constrict you, cause you to lose touch with your emotions, and diminish your spontaneity.

Protective Clothing for Caregivers

The use of psychological defenses is an integral part of caregiver survival. Caregiving is a process of adjusting to stress and loss: the loss of the person you knew and the loss of the way things used to be. As such, it can be thought of as a grieving process, the purpose of which is to relinquish the dreams and beliefs associated with a loved one. Letting go of your credo or your defenses is frightening. It raises the question, "If I can't have that which was central to my existence, and I let go of it, where do I go now? What will I do now?" (Moses, 1992).

Faced with the bleakness of a world turned upside down, the caregiver has three options. One option is to avoid pain by *distancing yourself* from it. Distancing or isolating yourself from psychological pain calls forth defenses, the most basic of which is *denial*. There are several aspects of denial, all of which are invoked to make the awfulness of what is happening cease to exist.

- Initially denial can be related to warding off the reality of what is happening. ("Go away. I will not acknowledge that this exists.") When Trisha, Fred's daughter, asked him if he had noticed that Ruth seemed to be forgetting things, he said, "No."

- On another level, denial can allow the caregiver to ignore the significance, or meaning, of what is happening. ("Go away, I don't understand the implication of what is happening.")
  Trisha: Have you noticed that Mom needs to have things repeated more often now?
  Fred: Yes, we all become a little forgetful when we get older.

- Last, denial can help avoid the feelings associated with what is happening. ("Go away. I won't let what is happening touch me.")
  Trisha: I know it's hard for you with Mom needing so much help.
  Fred: Yes, but I can manage. We'll get through this fine. Didn't I always take care of your mother?

Denial is not necessarily unhealthy. It can grant a reprieve, allowing you to gather strength and resources. Denial is unhealthy only when you can't get beyond it and when it becomes your only way of coping with the stresses of caregiving.

A second option, or reaction, to pain and anxiety is to choose to *anesthetize yourself*. This can take the form of becoming over-involved in the details of caregiving, becoming so busy doing the job that there is no time to feel. Alternately, there is numbing one's self with substance (i.e. drugs and alcohol). This becomes a never-ending course, because when the substance wears off, the pain returns.

The third option is to *grieve*, to let go of the dreams and expectations of the past, and to accept the sadness, anger, frustration and loss. The grieving process necessitates acknowledging painful emotions that defy predictability and control. However, the grieving process prepares us for the future ---- to be in touch with ourselves, to go forward, to change and to reinvest in others.

5

TRANSITION

David Wolpe, in his book, *In Speech And In Silence*, concisely describes the duress endured by families of loved ones with life-threatening or irreversible illness.

> *A long illness resolves to episodes. At each step along the way, it seems to move forward ---- to get past this problem would be total triumph. Long range thinking is too difficult; stamina is the gift of a day, not years or even weeks. "Dear God, let me make it through this day," is the prayer of one in pain. So there are phases; there is the shock of beginning, which gives way to the long waiting, the anguish of impotence when all one can hope for is the resource of a loved one, the unfathomable artistry of the doctor, the grace of God, if God dwells in those small, forlorn hospital chapels.* ---- Wolpe, 1992

At the onset of a life-threatening condition, the hospital is the center of life. The routine of the hospital becomes the outline into which family members structure their existence: The time of the doctor's visit, the chair next to the bed, the hand stroked for response, the observations made by the nurse, the flutter of an eye, the coolness of a brow, the elevator that makes too many stops, the chapel where you pray.

April 1988. Becca sat beside Brian as he drifted in and out of coma. Sometimes he seemed ready to awaken and then was lost to her again. His life was still painfully unguaranteed. She busied her mind with details, reminding herself of the questions she wanted to ask the doctors and the nuances of change she wanted to report. She rallied herself and then called on God for strength.

"You must be strong, too." She murmured to the unresponsive Brian. "Fight, and don't let go."

Becca had learned that early. It was part of being in control, not being weak, and doing whatever was necessary.

In the quiet of the hospital room, it occurred to Becca that Brian was not as tenacious as she. As usual, she struggled with how to guide him to follow her course. She worried that his "free spirit" would not have the perseverance to pull him through. She wanted to teach him how to be strong, but she knew that first she would have to give, in order to get.

"I was not always strong," she said to her "sleeping" son (confessions made easily to ears that could not quite hear).

"When I was four, my mother got a job as a secretary at Litt's. I had to go to a day care center. There were many children at the center, and after the first visiting day, my mother could not stay with me.

"The other children did not play with me. Some took toys from me. One hit me on the foot with a block. I was lonely. I wanted to go home.

"The second day, I told my mother that I did not want to go back, but she said I would like it better when I got used to it. When we got there, my mother had to hurry to leave. Mrs. Crane, the teacher, saw that I was crying and took me by the hand.

"Carolyn Shippen stuck her tongue out at me and grinned. The other kids saw it and laughed. I knew that I would not show tears again. I would not cry for my mother."

Now Becca longed to cry, to cry to someone to make it better. She prayed that if, by some mishap, she could not save Brian and if he could not save himself, God would intervene and be merciful.

Changes and Adjustments

With the passing of the crisis, whether a traumatic injury or an ominous prognosis, efforts begin to adjust to life that will not be the same.

As time passes, the chronic illness of a family member creates confusion by increasing the number of roles and responsibilities of the caregiver. Roles in families are established over the course of many years. They become associated with a person and with his or her function in the household. Adjusting to changes in roles and responsibilities can be especially stressful if the caregiver has trouble relinquishing old expectations and old ways of dealing with the patient. Caregivers who continue to treat loved ones as they were before ---- that is, as if nothing has changed ---- are at risk for frustration and disappointment.

In the marital relationship, for example, goals, expectations, responsibilities and roles evolve over time. When one spouse becomes chronically ill, the relationship is seriously disrupted. The caregiver comes to feel no longer married to the same person. Feelings of loss and loneliness occur due to the change in the partner with whom dreams, experiences and decision-making were shared. Frequently there is a loss of intimacy and physical contact. Disruption of the couple's sexual relationship is, in part due to the change in the patient's sexual behavior and sexual interest. Caregivers also find themselves unable to be intimate with someone with whom they have taken on a parental role and with whom they can no longer communicate feelings and thoughts. Fatigue and depression in the caregiver also contribute to a lack of interest and diminished sexual desire.

> *August 1990.* Finally, in the evening, Fred found time to fold the laundry. He laid it out on the bed, intending to put it away after emptying the dishwasher. Ruth had been watching television but wandered into the bedroom.
>
> He called in to her, "I'll be in as soon as I get the dishwasher emptied."
>
> He heard the music from the bedroom. Ruth was playing old songs on the stereo.
>
> "Stars shining bright above you... da, da, da, da, da... whisper I love you."
>
> He walked into the bedroom to check her. Laundry was strewn haphazardly around, as if she had been looking for something. There, turning and whirling in her bra and slip, was Ruth. Seeing him, she stretched out her arms in an invitation to a dance.
>
> He could not move toward her and found himself caught, not knowing whether to laugh or flee.

Change Stresses the Relationship

The need to take on new responsibilities and learn new skills comes at a time when the caregiver's resources and energy are already strained. Additional responsibilities may also be anxiety-arousing and distasteful.

Patients with dementia frequently exhibit childlike and inappropriate behavior. These behaviors may be embarrassing for the caregiver, thus making it difficult for the caregiver to respond to the loved one in a positive way. The decline in the patient's mental capacity requires that the caregiver assume a "parental" role, which both the caregiver and the patient may resist. For the patient it highlights the inability to function independently. For the caregiver it means an increased need to be supportive and in charge. These changes for the caregiver may precipitate stress, anger, and resentment about the decline of the mutuality in the relationship.

In *marital relationships* these negative and resentful feelings create caregiver guilt. As feelings change, the quality of the relationship changes, and even tender feelings are not those of a marital relationship.

Muriel Lezak (1978) wrote about the special problems of caregivers adjusting to living with a spouse with brain pathology. The caregiver lives in a kind of "social limbo," not actually having a partner for social activities, but not being able to seek out another partner. Furthermore, while there has been an actual loss of the *person* one married, society neither recognizes nor approves of a grieving or mourning process while the patient is alive. The caregiver cannot leave. He or she remains bound by past ties, present responsibilities, and guilt ---- while many of the connections which sustained the marriage have been lost.

When a son or daughter becomes caregiver for a *parent*, roles are reversed. Children who historically turned to a parent for guidance and support may experience feelings of abandonment and sadness in the face of the parent's deteriorating mental capacities. Even for the adult child, the loss of the parenting person and the change in responsibilities force a role change. Ambivalence is felt when the adult child begins making decisions for the parent. Anger and conflict occur if the parent does not cooperate or agree with the decisions that are made.

Somewhat different adjustments are required when the caregiver is the parent of an *adult impaired child*. Caregivers of cognitively impaired adult children sadly anticipate continued dependency of their children. In addition to the caregiver's anticipation of permanent responsibility for the adult child, there is the sorrow of realizing that one will have to continue to minister to a child who will never quite be grown up.

> *October 1989.* Brian had a well-coordinated team helping with rehabilitation. While it had been a year since his release from Booth Rehabilitation Center, he still required supervision, even in his daily routine.
>
> Between his physical therapy and cognitive rehabilitation, the days were tightly scheduled. When a member of the team was not working with Brian at home, Becca transported him back to Booth's outpatient department for the therapies that could be obtained only there.
>
> Brian now had good use of his hands and arms, although he continued to have problems with balance and coordination. Most impairing was his difficulty in expressing himself verbally. He often could not find the words or put them together in correct syntax. Frequently, when having trouble expressing himself, he would get angry. Sometimes he was just moody, and Becca felt isolated from him.
>
> Perhaps he was depressed. Perhaps it was something he just could not find the words to express. Becca tried to give him space, careful not to recreate the pattern of her being intrusive and directive. She struggled, though, with concern for a son who was, once again, a child, but who would not be able to tolerate another assault to his manhood.
>
> The fact that he continued to make progress kept Becca afloat, but it was clear that he would never be able to live independently. She tried not to become obsessed with concerns for his future.

Finally, for the caregiver of an adult child, there is anxiety about how care will continue for the adult child if something happens to the caregiver.

Change Stresses the Whole Family

The above noted role changes have repercussions for the extended family. Extended family relationships are strained as energy and attention are directed to the patient and away from other family members. Resentment, feelings of abandonment, conflict and tension grow over time. As family members' needs are compromised, they become less and less able to mutually support each other, and distance develops. Relatives outside the immediate family often find it painful to watch the deterioration of a loved one and, therefore, stay away. Similarly, caregivers, because of their intense involvement with the patient, increasingly withdraw and isolate themselves from the world.

The Physical Costs of Caregiving

The stress of providing chronic care has been linked to the development or intensification of physical complaints and even the weakening of the immune system. Caregivers frequently complain of headache, stomach distress, muscle aches, insomnia and other symptoms.

November 1989. Becca lay awake next to Tom, resenting his ability to fall asleep, yet relieved that he was sleeping and asking nothing of her. She realized that they had not touched for months.

Earlier that evening, they had argued. Tom had stayed late at work to finish a project, and consequently Becca had missed her book club meeting (the one escape she allowed herself) because she could not leave Brian alone.

They had quarreled about responsibility for Brian. Tom looked sheepish and complained, like an abandoned child, about his needs going unmet. Becca was angry that he could bring up his needs when her own needs routinely went unnoticed.

Now, as she lay in bed, still wound up from the day, she thought about tomorrow and the meeting with the team. She must remember to tell them that Brian was not progressing well with the new leg exercise. She shifted, trying to settle in. Chronic fatigue itself, as well as the inability to give up the day, interfered with her ability to sleep. *Becca, if you rest, will he slip between your fingers?* The silence of the night was like a blanket... and finally, sleep, as the morning hours neared.

Fatigue, a common caregiver phenomenon, potentially lowers physical resistance and makes the caregiver more susceptible to illness, as do poor eating habits and poor sleeping habits. The physical labor exerted in caregiving (such as lifting and carrying) puts strain on the knees, hips and back, and can aggravate preexisting conditions such as arthritis and osteoporosis. Possible links between the stress of caregiving and development of more serious illness including heart disease, high blood pressure and cancer are being researched.

Too often caregiving requires handling countless new responsibilities in the absence of good support. For respite, a caregiver may turn to a maladaptive stress reliever, such as drugs or alcohol. Prior use of prescription drugs or social drinking may slowly intensify to the point of dependency or substance abuse.

December 1989. Nora got home late from the hospital on the day that Glenn went in for his second round of chemotherapy. At 6:15 when she would normally have greeted him with a martini, she poured one for herself. She sat down, missing the comfort of sharing his day with a before-dinner drink. She poured a drink for him anyway, trying to recreate his presence. She drank her martini and then drank his. Why waste it? She felt a little lighter.

After that when she came home from the hospital, she continued to have drinks for both of them. In time, one more to help her get to sleep. Even after Glenn came home from the hospital she would slip out to the living room for a brandy before she went to bed.

In March, when the CAT Scan revealed that the tumor was no longer shrinking, Nora felt the fear again. She went home, closed the door, and went directly to the liquor cabinet. The tartness of the brandy licked her throat, and the warmth branched out in her chest like crimson, velvet fingers, bringing calm.

6

THE EMOTIONAL ASPECTS
OF CAREGIVING

*The man I love is but a shell of himself. It's a tease. He is there,
but not there. He is the same, and yet he is different. He is a
member of our family, and yet not the same member of the
family. How will I cope? How will I keep from becoming bitter,
lonely, and withdrawn? What will happen to us? How will I
live a life that will be fulfilling and meaningful?*

---- Doernberg, 1986

These concerns, written by caregiver Myra Doernberg, reflect a
host of emotions including fear, confusion, frustration,
depression, anger and guilt.

Human beings are intellectual, spiritual, physical and
emotional creatures. Caregivers accept the need to use their
intellect, expend physical energy, and have faith. They are,
however, often unprepared for the range and intensity of the
emotional challenge. As individuals, caregivers differ in their
emotional reactions. Some factors which affect how the caregiver
deals with the emotional challenge include the pre-existing
personality, the ability to cope with stress, personal circumstances

at the time a loved one becomes ill, emotional stamina, the nature of the relationship between the caregiver and the loved one, and the attitude toward the role of caregiving. Although some caregivers are able to cope with their feelings fairly well, all experience emotional stress.

Subsequent to acknowledging the facts and the implications of chronic illness, coping requires a recognition of the accompanying emotions. The key to coping effectively with feelings is *modulation*. To modulate is neither to suppress or deny feelings, nor to allow them to rampage and overwhelm. It is the ability to express feeling within an appropriate range.

Typically the first emotional responses to trauma are fear and denial. Following that, there is no orderly, predictable way of responding emotionally. An emotion may be expressed and seemingly dealt with, only to surface again at a later date, in a new context.

Fear

Fear is the immediate response to disaster. Fear brings confusion, a sense of unreality and numbness, and an inability to concentrate. Emotionally, fear is a general state of alarm, analogous to the physical shock following trauma. Fear is the panic that Becca felt as she hung up the telephone.

Denial

After shock has subsided, denial is the prevailing reaction to life-threatening illness. During the initial stage of denial, there is an attempt to expect and hope that things will return to normal. Accompanying this may be fantasies of miraculous recovery. When reality is too threatening, denial is a temporary reprieve which provides time to gather resources in order to deal with the situation.

Denial continues either until you are strong enough to deal with the stress, or until repeated crises and affronts cause denial to break down.

September 1990. The months passed and Glenn became progressively more frail. Nora had more and more difficulty pretending he would get better and that things would return to the way they had been. He was increasingly dependent and needful of her care; her needs were no longer primary.

Nora found that Glenn's dependency made her anxious. Tasks seemed endless. She helped him dress, she carried in the groceries by herself, she climbed into the attic for the winter comforters, she rushed to close all of the windows during a sudden rain shower.

She was tired, and then even more tired — unsure of herself and stretched too thin. Fatigue and apprehension replaced security and comfort.

Anxiety

As denial breaks down, anxiety ---- previously warded off ---- is now felt. Anxiety is the fear of being unprotected, unsafe and abandoned. It also evolves out of fear of losing love or being deprived of needs. Serious illness in a loved one may evoke anxiety about your safety. It elicits the thought, *It could happen to me.* It touches the previously repressed, now frighteningly aroused, awareness of our human vulnerability and mortality.

February 1991. Nora attended a support group for families of cancer patients at the hospital. She listened to others whose plights seemed more serious than hers and Glenn's. She was comforted that Glenn's illness did not seem as life-threatening as the others.

When Glenn's condition began to sound like the others', Nora stopped going to the group.

She mentioned to Dr. Radick that she was having difficulty sleeping and was worried that she would not be able to care for Glenn if he got very sick.

Dr. Radick assured her that he and the hospital staff would be there in emergencies and could get Glenn into the hospital quickly. He noticed the tension in her face and recommended some form of stress reduction for her.

Sonnie, Nora's old college roommate, suggested a relaxation group, Transcendental Meditation.

Nora went.

She listened intently to the instructor *who could make things better.*

The leader described how they were to allow their minds to settle down while sitting comfortably with their eyes closed. "The goal is pure awareness, being awake without thought."

Nora resolutely took a deep breath and concentrated.

"The means toward attaining this state is the use of *mantra,*" a sound in thought, "which is an effective way of disengaging from everyday thinking to quiet mental activity" (Maharishi Mahesh Yogi, 1970).

Each individual who practices Transcendental Meditation selects a mantra that is suitable for himself. Many people select the mantra, "Om," which has been called a "universal sound," with good effects for those who chant it aloud or silently.

Nora sat cross-legged on the floor in yoga position. She glanced around, having trouble settling herself down. Her agitation interfered with her ability to bend herself to the suggestion of the teacher.

Next to her sat a man whose lips mouthed the sound, "Om." Nora watched as he repeated it, and the "Om" became "One" in her perception. Her stomach twisted with the dread of aloneness which would be hers if Glenn died.

She felt herself vault up and flee from the room.

Run from the healer, run from the fear, run from the silence. But don't run away. You are the caregiver.

And as a caregiver, you become deluged with anxieties which are associated with concerns about the outlook for your loved one, your own ability to handle the situation, and your own future. These fears, connected to real dilemmas, build and intensify the dread associated with the awful sense that everything is not going to be O.K. You may begin to feel overwhelmed and fearful that your own survival is being threatened.

This intense anxiety touches the security of one's existence and, paradoxically, leads to the "unsolvable, existential dilemma," noted by Ken Moses, "How can I get out of this life alive?" (1992).

Initially, anxiety can be paralyzing. Soon, however, you realize that it's necessary to mobilize, to adjust and change, to marshal your resources. You expect your interventions to alleviate the situation, and are not prepared to be frustrated in your efforts.

Frustration

There *is* frustration, however. Frustration associated with the decline of the patient's abilities. Frustration when annoying behaviors of the patient are not amenable to change. Frustration when the patient cannot or will not cooperate. Frustration in trying to communicate with a loved one, in trying to understand the needs of a loved one, and in trying to reason with a loved one who has compromised cognitive ability. Frustration in offering help which is rejected or resisted. Frustration associated with feelings of helplessness when the needs and demands of the patient increase in the absence of improvement. Finally, there is frustration when you feel powerless to change what has or will happen.

December 1991. Fred devised an orderly routine for dressing Ruth. It helped him feel organized and more in control. His hope was that Ruth would follow the pattern he established, thus solving one area of difficulty.

He thought it out in a systematic way. Right side, left side, arm up, arm down. He even imagined a rhythm and precision to it. Fred's way. Plan, order, effort, work it out. *No, Fred. Not this time.* Ruth perceived no pattern, followed no order. She jerked and resisted and never learned the routine, even when he was leading. And combing her hair and brushing her teeth were a nightmare.

Disappointment ---- and frustration ---- will result from unrealistic expectations of the loved one; expecting either too much or too little. Frequently there is frustration associated with unrealized hopes and in looking for signs of improvement or validation from others of progress that is not really there.

January 1992. When Ruth developed some problems with balance, Dr. Mellman ordered a new CAT Scan.

Fred wheeled Ruth into the medical center and, after registering, they went to wait in X-ray. Dr. Conner passed by and turned around when Fred called him. He had run some tests on Ruth earlier in the year.

"How are you?," he asked, addressing them both.

"Ruthie, tell the doctor how you are."

Silence.

"Here, show him the pictures." He pulled out the pictures that Trisha had recently sent of their grandchildren.

"Tell the doctor who they are," he coaxed her, hoping that she could point them out and recognize them as she had done the day before. She did not speak.

Resentment

The restrictions associated with caregiving itself can be embittering. Caregivers feel trapped as their lives change and their hopes for the future are thwarted.

> *Fall 1971.* "Woody!"
>
> His mother calling him from the kitchen. He knew what would follow.
>
> "Can ye' give me a lift gettin' up from this chair?"
>
> It was 8:30 in the evening. She would want him to put away the dishes. Tired from the day himself, he expected that she'd call him in as she gathered herself to the task, both of them knowing, though, that he'd be doing it. Now he was at her call because, of course, he could not let her. He was irked at the predictability of the game.
>
> "You know I'd do it. You didn't have to start." As usual he tried to avoid looking at her. The mingling of anger and pain, he knew, would circle in his stomach at the picture of her, weak and short of energy at day's end. The picture was quickly accompanied by a flashback to years ago, the way she used to prevail and make the space around her resonate to her will.
>
> Now her call wove around and through him, but it brought pity and resentment. It made him want to flee, to get in his car and drive off and never look back. He wanted to find a place of his own and not have her there.

The loss of previous lifestyle, the absence of hope that things will get better, leads to resentment. Resentment and loss of hope are wearing, and caregivers may get angry at themselves for not coping better. Individuals who believe that hard work can make things better and give them control find that hard work is no guarantee of progress. The breakdown of the myth, "If I work hard enough, good things will happen," leaves the caregiver feeling helpless.

In some instances, other family members and the community of the caregiver become the target for anger. Caregivers may feel that they have to put on a facade of coping well, as other people compliment them on the wonderful job they are doing. This makes it more likely that friends and other family members will not offer needed help and support.

December 1989. Becca felt that she had to make all the decisions about Brian's treatment by herself. She met with the rehabilitation team regularly and reported to them on what seemed to be working and how Brian was progressing at home.

Tom, in passing, would ask how the meeting went or if Brian was having a good day. Once in a while he offered to go to a meeting in her place, but Becca did not trust him to give the team an accurate report.

However, she resented Tom's willingness to let her take care of things, because it left her little time for herself. She was trapped by her need for control and exactness, but maddened by the paradoxical loss of control of her life that resulted from her need for vigilance.

Family members who give advice but are not involved in the burden of caregiving on a daily basis are seen as intrusive or lacking understanding. This also generates resentment.

You may experience intense and recurring anger toward professionals and institutions who fail (or appear to fail) to provide needed information and assistance. Caregivers complain about unanswered questions, lack of sympathy, and roadblocks to getting needed services. The perceived lack of help increases the burden of caregiving and fosters anger in the already overstressed caregiver.

Anger

Caregivers may be able to acknowledge that they are frustrated, anxious, or even in denial. They are, however, unprepared for anger.

Anger is a strong emotion. It is displeasure, aroused by feelings of being wronged, or by feelings of being treated unjustly. Anger is a typical reaction to frustration. It is easiest to acknowledge when it is felt to be justified.

Although it is not abnormal to experience anger when frustrated, caregiver anger is often followed by guilt. This is likely the case if you feel that it isn't "right" to be angry with an impaired loved one who is not in control of him/herself. Additionally it's uncomfortable to express anger if you have always viewed it in connection with impulsive or unacceptable behavior. Your anger, therefore, may be suppressed, and create tension and/or depression.

Expressing anger is mentally and physically draining, but it is also tiring to expend energy and effort to suppress anger.

Patients with cognitive impairments behave in ways that are irritating and wearing on your tolerance. Repeating the same question, increasing demandingness, compromised reasoning ability, impulsive and/or inappropriate behavior all tend to provoke.

> *September 1990.* Ruth asked again, "Fred, I would like to know what you will be making us for dinner, dear."
>
> "Ruthie, you already had your dinner."
>
> "I did? What did I have? I don't remember having dinner." She looked puzzled, as if disbelieving, but was quiet.
>
> A few moments later he passed her on his way to the den. She was sitting at the dining room table.
>
> "I'm feeling like I should have a bit of dinner, hmmmm." She crooned after him.
>
> Over his shoulder, "Flounder filets, remember?"
>
> Of course she didn't, and looked at him more insistently. He tried to contain his irritation.

Caregivers also find it annoying when they are trying to be helpful and are rebuffed. At times it is difficult to separate being angry with *the patient* and being angry at *the patient's behavior.* Caregivers do not always recognize that patients' impairments limit their control over their behavior. In addition, the desire to have the loved one be as before interferes with accepting the loved one's limitations. This can result in negative exchanges.

Expressing anger appropriately is a challenge. Denying or displacing the anger does not work, for it builds up and increases the potential for uncontrolled outbursts.

> *March 1992.* Ruth had always liked to joke. Over the years, Fred had come to reconcile himself to her fooling, although he tended to be more serious.
>
> Now she resisted as he tried to put her arm through the sleeve of a clingy, white blouse. She stiffened, then wriggled her arm like a child, but her curly grey hair belied the childish motion.
>
> Fred felt the frustration and anger rise as he held her arm with one hand and again tried to maneuver her hand through the sleeve.

She looked him right in the eye and flipped her right shoulder in opposition to his hold.

He sighed heavily, tensed, and clenched his teeth. His hands fastened on her, grabbing angrily as he lost control and shook her and shook her again. Her nostrils flared and her lip quivered like a child recoiling from the sting of a slap. Then she stood still, immobilized by fear.

Fred sat down, bewildered by his unexpected release of emotion.

Soldier in the battle of injustice, who waves his "arms" in frustration and pierces his dream in his frenzy.

If you do not acknowledge anger and do not allow a tempered expression of frustration, the anger builds. Caregivers who cannot step away from the situation, even briefly, in order to regain composure, are at risk for an unmodulated release of anger. Any such loss of control, though, is unacceptable and leads to guilt.

Guilt

If we feel that we have done something wrong, behaved badly (like getting angry when we shouldn't), or have been neglectful, we feel guilty. Guilt is the **M**onolithic **F**ractionator of all emotions.

March 1992. "Damn!" Fred looked down. His eyes caught the two bluish marks on Ruth's upper arm. "Damn!" He glanced to see if she had followed his gaze. Would she understand, anyway?

Small ellipses mirrored the shape of his thumbs and middle fingers, which had grabbed her when he shook her.

Again he looked and his gaze caught hers. What was it in the grey-blue of her eyes. Fear? Disappointment? Now her irises darkened. Was she afraid of him? The absence of her words made him try to read her eyes.

Speak to me with your eyes. I'm sorry, he silently pleaded.

Caregiver guilt is associated with an action, thought, feeling or belief about the loved one. It is keenly felt because it affects self-esteem and the sense of self-worth. Guilt can lead to self-doubt, and can immobilize decision-making. It is an emotional drain and can result in overindulgence and over-protectiveness of the loved one.

The role of caregiver provides ample opportunity for feeling guilty. Many caregivers feel that they are not being nurturant enough if they take time out for themselves. Therefore, they are reluctant to leave the loved one alone.

Guilt can result if tender and needy feelings toward the loved one are replaced by a custodial attitude. Anger toward the person who cannot, or will not, learn or perform as before is quickly followed by guilt when you acknowledge it is not the patient's fault.

As your loved one's condition deteriorates you may lose respect for him or her. This can also precipitate guilt.

If your relationship with the patient prior to illness was not particularly good, you may experience regret and have concerns about whether you will be able to make it up to the patient. Looking back, caregivers often blame themselves and question whether they could have done something to prevent the loved one's becoming ill. You may wonder whether you are taking good enough care to prevent a worsening of the condition. The caregiver who asks God what s/he has done for this to happen is not asking for a theological explanation, but for reassurance that s/he is a good person. As a caregiver you must accept that bad things happen and you are not to blame.

The very nature of caregiving is alien and unappealing for some caregivers. They may not be basically nurturing people and may be uncomfortable with the role.

> *June 1972.* "Woody!"
> The call... just as he was on the way out.
> "I'll be needin' a few things from th' market, if ye' going out again."
> Again! It was Saturday afternoon and he hadn't been out yet. He was looking forward to meeting Karen and spending the afternoon with her.
> Megan, so lucky, had a life of her own — just married and living halfway across the country. Away from Mam's "needin." How was he the one who ended up with Mam, when, from the time he was a boy, he had only been waiting for the day when he could escape?

You may, like many caregivers, have thought about abandoning the caregiving role. And the thought may lead you to feel that you are selfish and are not doing what is expected. The expectations of others regarding the caregiver's responsibilities combine with your own guilt, and the desire to escape is quickly albeit temporarily pushed out of mind.

Caregivers have difficulty watching their loved ones lead compromised, often uncomfortable, lives. While they typically live in dread of something awful happening to the loved one, thoughts do intrude about the death of the loved one as a release for both of them. The conflict arising from these thoughts results in feelings of shame and guilt.

> *August 1991.* Nora stood by Glenn's hospital bed. He had just returned from a round of chemotherapy and was sleeping. She looked at him. Strange how different he looked. Older, maybe. So still. Almost as if dead. She wondered what it would be like if he were dead, and her mind wandered.
>
> *She saw the funeral gathering. Tears, her own. She would indulge in crying. Faces, she imagined, gathering around. Arms to console her.*
>
> Now she felt guilty because she had imagined him dead.

The guilt of the caregiver. The wish for relief. The wish to be consoled, cared for. So unacceptable. The wish so quickly denied.

Isolation

The feeling of isolation is another consequence of caregiving. Caregivers frequently feel that other people do not understand what they are going through. Often they are too busy and confined by the demands of caregiving to keep up social contacts. If, however, they don't make strong efforts to have time and space for themselves, their lives are likely to be consumed by caregiving.

Fatigue also interferes with the maintenance of external contacts. The loneliness which results from isolation is intensified by the loss of communication and sharing with the loved one. The loved one may be physically present but no longer able to understand and express thoughts. In some instances, as the illness progresses, the loved one eventually even loses the ability to recognize the caregiver.

Jealousy

February 1990. Jealousy further isolated Becca from her family and friends. Becca had never thought of herself as a jealous person, but now she felt resentment toward friends who appeared to have time and freedom. She longed for the normality of everyday things. She envied friends for their unhurried trips to the supermarket, their chats over coffee, and the luxury of their unplanned spare time.

It is not uncommon for caregivers to feel jealous toward others whose lives appear unperturbed, still whole and fulfilling. It is also normal to feel jealousy or resentful feelings toward the patient, who appears to be receiving a lot of attention and caring.

Depression

Depression and grief are similar, in that both have their genesis in loss. Loss is typically followed by depression, and the loss associated with a deteriorating condition leads to depression.

Depression, then, is a normal response to loss, but it can become an impairment if it is chronic and interferes with functioning. Depression can be evidenced in both physical and emotional symptoms. Physical symptoms of depression include appetite and sleep disturbance, slowness of speech and thought, and fatigue. The interplay of fatigue and depression in caregiving in cyclical. Caregiving is in itself fatiguing, which leads to feelings of depression; and then being depressed makes the caregiver feel more fatigued.

Research findings have reported that one in three of all caregivers have experienced at least one episode of depression, in contrast to one in five for the U.S. population as a whole.

Emotionally, depressed individuals experience feelings of emptiness, sadness and pessimism. It is the feeling of pessimism, that the future is bleak and without meaning, that turns sadness into depression. In addition, the depressed person may suffer from impaired self-worth, inhibition, and a withdrawal from life's activities. Extreme despondency can result in suicidal thoughts and wishes.

Caregivers who resist ventilating their anger on the patient or on others, hold it in and therefore experience stress.

January 1992. By January, Glenn was very weak and very sick. Nora did just about everything for him. She helped him dress, walk and shower, and she even moved his glass closer at dinner so that he did not have to stretch.

This was an enormous change for Nora, whose family had never let her do much for herself or anyone else. She, who had no practice in making choices or taking care, now found herself with all the responsibilities. In the face of her self-doubt, she was rattled by her duties as caregiver but, nonetheless, kept busy. Run to the market, run to the bank, run to get home... time to run away. *But you cannot go. You are the caregiver. You must stay.*

One morning when she was helping Glenn dress, he growled at her. "I can do it myself."

She started back, surprised by this new aspect, which replaced the gentle, accepting Glenn. She was hurt by his outburst and then depressed because she was trying so hard and he did not seem to notice. She could not permit herself to get angry with him or even tell him how hard she was trying.

Grief

Grief is an emotional reaction to the loss of someone or something that is an important part of oneself.

Grief is a normal reaction to loss. While grief is typically associated with loss through death, there are other grief-worthy losses: loss of a relationship through divorce; loss of a friend; loss of a job; loss of a home; loss of self-esteem; loss of the role of parent, spouse, or child; loss of a belief; loss of a physical part of one's self; loss of identity; developmental loss, such a mid-life crisis or retirement; and loss of a dream.

Grief is the price we must be prepared to pay if we connect. If we make significant attachments, we take the chance that at some point we may have to grieve. Grief is pain expressed internally through thoughts and feelings and felt through anger, sadness, despair and even physical symptoms.

Caregivers, who deal with losses that occur during chronic illness, grieve. Their grief, though, differs from the grief brought about by the death of a loved one. In death, there is finality, and grief is followed by mourning. Caregiver grief goes on and on.

June 1990. It was like mourning, except she saw no end to it. Becca would see college boys driving with their girlfriends or young men with families, and she would think, *That will never be Brian.*

She would have to give up the dream of Brian as an independent adult with a family of his own. With that went the hope that someday he would understand her better and know what "parent" meant.

There were so many dreams that she had to give up about Brian. So much she felt was lost. So much they would never have.

Letting go is the ultimate pain of grief. Grieving for a chronically ill loved one begins before the actual physical loss occurs. The slow, psychological deterioration of the loved one results in increasing emotional separation. Although the caregiver may be more and more involved with the physical condition of the loved one, there is less opportunity to be connected psychologically and to be involved with the loved one as a person.

1992. In April, Glenn returned to the hospital to die. At times he did not recognize her. The growth which had begun in his stomach had metastasized to his brain and played havoc with his ability to think, understand, communicate and be awake. He never said her name, but occasionally would answer her touch when she pressed his hand.

She was drowning in her fear of being without him and in the alcohol which by now had become a standard part of getting through both day and night.

Concerned friends would ask about how Glenn was and about how he was doing. "Fine." If she allowed herself to consider an answer, she would be driven further into the numbness of alcohol.

Now she sat by the bed, smoothing the wrinkled white sheet near his shoulder, trying to bring some tidiness into his world. He moved and his eyes flickered open. She searched his eyes for recognition and connection, but they were a cloudy, unfamiliar color. *He must be in there.*

"Speak to me with your eyes." Her voice was less than a whisper. His lids opened, but then his eyes closed again.

"Glenn, can you hear me?" she ventured with more assurance. *Words lost. Mine to you, unheard. Yours to me. Unsaid.* "Speak to me with your eyes." *We know each other well.* And when he did not respond, "I love you," her voice sought to reach him.

When seeing a dying animal a man feels a sense of horror: substance similar to his own perishing before his eyes. But when it is a beloved and intimate human being that is dying, besides this horror at the extinction of life, there is a severance, a spiritual wound, which like a physical wound is sometimes fatal and sometimes heals, but always aches and shrinks to any external touch.   ---- Tolstoy, 1942

It is not unusual, as the process of distancing and disconnecting is occurring, that caregivers wish for a painless release of the loved one through death. Caregivers may experience guilt about their growing emotional distance from the loved one. They may not be able to accept that in this time of intense turmoil, their feelings and reactions are normal.

While families of chronically ill patients begin the grieving process long before the death of their loved ones, few caregivers are prepared for the pain of the final loss.

April 13, 1992. Nora sat in the funeral director's wood-panelled office. She gathered her energy to focus on the details as they talked together, making arrangements. She was aware of nothing but the rhythm of his words and the patches of lighter colors against the brown walls of his office.

Then... Curious the things you notice. The long, white tips of the funeral director's fingernails as he took down family information. Long, for a man, she noted in the midst of intense pain. (Strange how the mind dances outside itself.) Odd. She speculated on what kind of person he could be as he maintained utmost control in this time of her pain. What was the connection between his long fingernails and the measured pace of his speech? Then in a spectroscopic second, Glenn's face, the blueness of his eyes, the ruddy tone of his skin, appeared off to the right in a visual image forty-five degrees above her head. Unscathed and whole for a moment, then gone. But he's gone. And then again the pain, deep under her ribs. All the preparing and knowing, but not prepared, and never really knowing.

7

COPING

All systems require fuel in order to function. The human system "caregiver" is fueled by support, information, caring, ingenuity, stamina and the commitment to help. The escalating needs of an impaired loved one deplete the caregiver's resources. Without rest, time out and refueling, the caregiver is at risk for malfunction.

How well the caregiver copes with a chronically ill loved one depends on several factors. These include the severity and demands of the illness, the extent of the caregiver's support system, and the degree of family cohesiveness. Receptivity to support and information and the caregiver's willingness to be concerned about his/her own well-being improve the ability to cope.

When you're a caregiver, it is important to balance the patient's needs with your own in order to avoid physical, emotional and financial exhaustion.

Caregivers need to be able to establish realistic expectations of themselves. This requires an acceptance of the limits of what one person can do for another, and an understanding of the relationship between caring for a loved one and caregiving. In being loving and concerned for another person, one shows caring. Caregiving, however, need not require total self-sacrifice and perfection.

To recognize and function within your limits does not diminish your value as a caregiver. Each caregiver has a limit on how much he/she is able to do.

Spring 1977. Woody is 25. He has stopped for a beer or two on his way home from work this Friday night. He is back living with Mam these past two years, after leaving in 1973.

Home close to 9:00 p.m., he comes into the apartment.

"Woody!"

Mother o' God. The woman was half cracked. Standing on the top step, arms waving, dressed up like a peacock out to a parade. Dressed for what, he wondered. He remembered what the doctor had said about MS coming from a loss of myelin insulation covering parts of the brain cells. Was she losing the "myelin" that held together all rhyme and reason in her head?

Then he remembered. She'd told him she had a party at the social club.

"Ye' selfish dog... "

Who was she calling a dog? She who, before, during and forever in MS, was the leader of the pack.

"Ye' go off to be with ye' pals knowin' I'd be needin' ye'." (Her voice took on more of the brogue when she became emotional.)

Off she went, grousin' as Pop used to say. Nowadays she was more likely to get riled up and cry or to be angry easier. She tended to react out of proportion. But that was the illness. Well, maybe this time she had a right — looking forward, as he knew her to be, to get to her get-together with her friends, and him coming home late.

Since living at home again, though, he found himself not so irritated at her, and he just couldn't get mad now — impossible, as he looked at her with that ridiculous hat with the fruit salad stapled to the front of it.

"O.K., O.K., sorry. I'll take you now if you still want. Better late than not at all."

Her lips pursed forward, teeth clenching in her cheeks, she narrowed her eyes and lanced her gaze at him.

"Ye' better hurry and help me down from here. The one time in twenty when I'm really needin' ye'."

He helped her down the steps and took her by the elbow, feeling surprisingly protective and nearly possessive of her.

"Yah, Mam, I know you need me more now. Used to make me mad, the extra chores and you calling me all the time and not being up to it yourself. But now we just will have mind each other's feelings and do the best we can and not wait for the impossible."

She looked at him. "Well, sure now. I know ye' done all ye' could, and I'm appreciatin' it. Of course I'm grateful to ye'. Ye've been right decent to ye' Mam."

Find Ways to Care for Yourself

The limits for each caregiver are determined by physical, emotional, financial and social factors. In recognizing these limits, be sure to acknowledge your need for private time allotted to doing anything that is appealing or meaningful to you.

Occasional self-indulgence is important in order to alleviate the exhaustion and energy loss which compromise the ability to provide good care. Proper nutrition, rest and exercise are necessary in order to maintain good health.

Physical exercise, whether mild or vigorous, is a good stress reducer and a source of renewed energy. Choose a sport that you can do well and that allows for socializing. Research has shown that exercise increases the secretion of endorphins ---- chemicals in the brain that promote a feeling of well-being ---- and thus reduces stress.

Relaxation techniques, such as meditation, yoga and imaging, also reduce stress and give a feeling of tranquility. To maximize the probability of following through on these interventions, they should be scheduled at the same time and place every day. A simple but effective relaxation procedure described by Benson (1975) and others is as follows:

A Simple Relaxation Procedure

1. Find a comfortable place — Sit with your head, arms, legs, neck, and back supported, with shoes off and clothes loosened.

2. Take a deep breath, hold it, and be aware of the muscle tension in your chest. Slowly exhale and notice the chest muscles relaxing. Repeat this.

3. Tense all your body muscles for a count of five and then slowly release. Feel the muscles relax. Keep your eyes closed while doing this.

4. Starting at the top of the head, allow all the remaining muscles to begin to relax. Tense and relax all muscles for 10 minutes.

5. Keep your eyes closed and imagine a real or fantasied peaceful place. Think of the images (visual, auditory, etc.) associated with the place and relax there.

6. Remain relaxed, imagining that you are in the peaceful place until it is time to return.

7. Return by counting from 1 to 5 slowly, to be in the present again by the count of five.

Time away, whether by oneself or in activities with others, provides the emotional and physical separation which helps the caregiver continue to be effective. Without time to separate and gain some distance, you're likely to become overwhelmed and feel helpless and emotionally stressed. Practically, then, caregivers need to make a list of activities they enjoy, decide what is feasible and how, and then implement their plans.

The actual formulation of a plan is important because, even with the best of intentions, without a concrete plan (a time, a place), you will find yourself doing some caregiving activity instead of taking time out. Time away, whether for brief or extended periods, requires planning in order for the caregiver to feel in control. The time away should be manageable. Therefore, it is recommended that you begin with an alternative arrangement for a short period of time. Gradually, as you and your and patient become comfortable with alternative care, the time away can be increased.

Suggestions for brief respites, from Karr (1992)* include:

- Taking a walk at twilight or early morning

- Sharing a fun experience with a friend

- Playing and visiting with grandchildren

- Playing favorite records or tapes

- Going to (car, home, flower) shows

- Deep breathing for relaxation

- Checking into a bed and breakfast for an overnight

- Meditating

- Building models

- Taking a bubble bath

- Regularly attending a senior center for lunch and recreation

- Taking photographs

- Repotting house plants

- Playing a favorite musical instrument

- Doing absolutely nothing

- Baking something special

- Finishing a project

- Taking a walk in a storm

- Going out on a boat

- Buying new clothes

---

*From Katherine L. Karr, *Taking Time for Me: How Caregivers Can Effectively Deal with Stress* (Amherst, NY: Prometheus Books). © 1992. Reprinted by permission of the publisher.

- Spending an afternoon in the library

- Working with a special craft or hobby

- Going out to eat specifically for the experience of being served

- Dressing up to go someplace special

- Watching children in the park

- Singing with a group

- Watching a sunset

- Joining a club or group activity

- Asking others for hugs

- Taking up bird watching

- Visiting a planetarium

- Writing letters to close friends

Humor is another potent antidote for stress. To be able to laugh at oneself and the world and see humor in adversity, will help you survive as a caregiver.

> *July 1990.* Brian kicked his foot against the base of the bathroom sink. Becca came in to the noise and found him.
> He looked so comical, shaving for the first time with a safety razor. He was trying to get between his upper lip and nose, but struggling to manage a right arm that would not bend accurately to his command.
> The shaving cream crept down to his elbow as he lathered, messed and re-lathered. He grimaced as he had to contort his arm to get the top hairs near his nose. Becca stifled a laugh, careful not to further agitate him, but he noticed and their glance met. Then simultaneously they burst into laughter, laughing hard while the shaving cream melted in small, white puddles in the sink.

Laughter is the godchild of love.

Build Your Support System

Your well-being as a caregiver also requires the establishment of a network of supports. Caregivers need to be nurtured in order to keep giving, to avoid becoming depleted. The support system is called upon for decisions and assistance. This can occur formally, as in a family meeting that is called to discuss a special issue, or informally with the caregiver asking for help as the needs arise.

The support system includes family and friends, as well as medical, legal, and social service professionals. It should be available not only for emergencies but also for the relief of ongoing daily stresses.

It is best to allow ill loved ones to do as much as possible for themselves. Impaired individuals do not lose all functions at one time. They need, as much as possible, to maintain a sense of independence, functionality, and the ability to advocate for themselves. You're encouraged not to be too quick to take over too much in an attempt to "rescue" your loved one.

When help *is* needed, don't try to do it all alone. Receptivity to support means accepting help from children, friends, in-laws, brothers, sisters and neighbors who can take over when you need time for yourself. Interested friends and relatives may feel shut out if you decline their offers of help and/or companionship. You may find yourself in self-imposed isolation if you avoid contact with others and do not make efforts to be involved in outside activities.

Caregiver isolation is also the result of the unfortunate development that others tend to distance from the caregiver. This reinforces the tendency toward self-reliance and pride in strength, which is an outgrowth of the American philosophical tradition of "rugged individualism."

Caregivers who resist external help must ask themselves why they do this, i.e. What do you believe about responsibility? What about your own needs versus the needs of others? When will it be time to consider your own priorities? What stops you from thinking about your own needs ---- Guilt? Fear? Need for approval? What are the consequences of continuing not to ask for support? A positive consequence is that the loved one's needs will likely be met, while the negative is that you are exhausted. If a central part of your identity is a need for approval, you must anticipate guilt feelings when you ask others for help and take time for yourself.

It is important to find someone who will listen, be sympathetic, and be an advocate for you. Sometimes this means seeking professional help or a support group.

You can assemble a list of resources that can be called upon for assistance by completing the chart on pages 58-59 (from Greutzner, 1992).

As human beings we are sustained by the mutuality of contact and support, which is part of relationships with others. From the earliest historical times, societies learned that individual survival (physical and emotional) depended on the support of the community. It is in aloneness that we experience anxiety about the finiteness of our existence. Particularly in times of stress, the need exists to reach beyond ourselves to connect with others and to hear and to be heard by others.

Rabbi Harold Kushner speaks to this special need in his discussion of the story of Job. In the Bible, when Job is in pain, friends come to comfort him. They give advice and try to respond to Job's question: "Why is God doing this to me?" But theological explanations are not what Job is seeking. "Job needed sympathy, more than he needed advice... he needed compassion, the sense that others felt his pain with him... he needed physical company, people sharing their strength with him... " (Kushner, 1983).

In the Jewish mourning ritual, the mourner recites a prayer, the Mourner's Kaddish, for eleven months after the death of the loved one. The prayer is recited during the synagogue service with other mourners. The bereaved feels consoled by others who share his or her feelings, and is comforted by the acceptance of the congregation.

In a similar way, support groups provide a commonality of experience in which many aspects of caregiving can be shared. Support groups are a source of practical information and of suggestions about how to manage the practical problems of caregiving. The groups also provide a milieu for the ventilation of feelings and frustrations, and the discussion of uncomfortable topics. Meeting people in a similar situation alleviates the feeling of aloneness and isolation, and provides an opportunity for socialization.

Appendix D provides a list of associations and support groups which have national offices, as sources of referral, as well as highly recommended reading materials.

PERSONAL/SOCIAL SUPPORT RESOURCES

Name:_____**Date:**_____

Using your own situation, check the most appropriate Personal/ Social Support to the right of each question. Try to check at least 3.

	Yourself	Spouse	Children	Other Family	Friends	Neighbors	Church	Pastor/Priest	Doctor	Other Professional	Support Group	Agency Staff	Other
1. Whom can you count on for transportation?													
2. Whom can you count on for financial help/decisions?													
3. Who helps most with household chores?													
4. Whom can you count on to get to appointments?													
5. Whom do you enjoy doing things with during the week?													
6. Whom can you count on in times of crisis?													
7. Whom can you count on to console you when you're physically sick?													
8. Whom can you count on to console you when you're upset?													
9. Whom would you seek out when you're frightened?													
10. Whom would you talk to when you're lonely?													
11. When you need to talk, whom can you count on to listen?													
12. With whom can you really be yourself?													
13. Whom do you trust completely?													

Using your own situation, check the most appropriate Personal/Social Support to the right of each question. Try to check at least 3.

	Yourself	Spouse	Children	Other Family	Friends	Neighbors	Church	Pastor/Priest	Doctor	Other Professional	Support Group	Agency Staff	Other
14. Who do you feel really appreciates you as a person?													
15. With whom do you have the most frequent contact?													
16. Whose advice are you most likely to accept?													
17. Who supports your independence the most?													
18. Who seems to understand you best?													
19. Who helps you to be honest with yourself?													
20. Who helps you keep a positive outlook?													
21. Whom do you enjoy being with the most?													
22. Who best understands your current situation?													
23. Who helps you work out your problems most?													
24. Who could temporarily take your place in caregiving?													
25. Whom do you trust regarding legal matters?													
26. Whom can you talk to about family problems?													

Get Help When You Need It

The need for assistance at times exceeds that which friends, family or groups can give. When these interventions are not enough, when time away is not renewing, and the caregiver feels just as stressed after taking time for herself, more comprehensive changes are necessary. It is important to recognize the warning signals that indicate that you are overwhelmed and in need of professional help. Indications of impaired ability to cope include (*Karr, 1992):

- Increased irritability
- Difficulty sleeping, awakening early, or excessive sleeping
- Loss of energy or zest for life
- Becoming increasingly isolated
- Feeling out of control, engaging in uncharacteristic actions or emotions (crying a lot, becoming shrill, focusing on petty things)
- Drinking too many caffeinated beverages or relying too much on nicotine and alcohol, sleeping pills, and other medications
- Changes in the body's normal functioning: a pounding heart, trembling hands, difficulties with digestion
- Becoming forgetful, having problems concentrating
- Becoming less interested in people or activities that were once a source of pleasure
- Eating significantly more or less than usual
- Engaging in compulsive behaviors: constantly cleaning and straightening up or fussing over small, unimportant details
- Becoming accident prone
- Inability to overcome feelings of depression or anxiety
- Denying physical or psychological symptoms: e.g., "There's nothing wrong with taking sleeping pills every night," or "Anybody would be depressed in my situation."
- Handling family members less gently or considerately than is customary
- Entertaining suicidal thoughts.

The type of help needed depends on the problem. It may be medical, psychological, or a self-help organization such as AA.

March 1992. The aides at the day care noticed the blue marks on Ruth's forearms. She shrank back when they attempted to lead her by the arm.

"Mr. Krasner," the director of the center said, "We have been noticing that Ruth seems nervous and agitated when the aides take her by the arm. Is everything all right at home?"

Fred was horrified by the implication and could only acknowledge how difficult it had become to care for Ruth. He was resistant to the suggestion that he might want to look into a nursing home for her.

About a month later, Dr. Mellman telephoned him. He said that the director of the day care center had contacted him regarding their concern that Ruth physically was not looking well. Dr. Mellman asked if Fred would come into the office to talk.

In the office, Dr. Mellman began by acknowledging the difficulty of the job Fred had been doing. "This is not a job a man expects to end up doing when he gets married. The cooking, cleaning, the washing for both of you. It takes its toll." He leaned back, drawing Fred forward to respond.

"They think that I abused her. They think that I hurt Ruth." Fred spoke and waited to see whether Dr. Mellman would concur.

"They telephoned me," was all he answered.

"I just get so frustrated when I'm trying to help her and she makes it difficult. I do everything I can for her. Most of the time she doesn't seem to even recognize me. She looks at me like I'm a stranger, or she'll call me Norm. That's her brother's name. She hardly talks, and when she does, it doesn't make sense. I talk to her. I... I plead with her. Sometimes she finally complies, but sometimes she's so stubborn. She'll close her mouth and lock her teeth on the spoon when I try to help her eat. And then I grab her... " Haltingly, "It wasn't supposed to be this way."

Dr. Mellman was gentle. "Like Mrs. Keller, I am concerned for Ruth — and for you. Perhaps it is time to consider that Ruth cannot be managed at home any longer. You seem exhausted and overwhelmed. Ruth's safety must be considered. An alternative living situation might be best for her now."

Fred nodded his head in assent.

Learn to Deal with Your Feelings

As a caregiver, to be able to deal with your emotions is an accomplishment apart from coping with the practical aspects of the role. Emotions are elusive callers. They are welcome to run rampant when they bring pleasure, but they are uncontrollable poachers when they elicit pain. We are, nonetheless, emotional ---- as well as physical, intellectual and spiritual ---- beings.

Our parents teach us how to take care of ourselves physically. In school we learn how to use our intellect. In our places of worship we find God and our spiritual sense. Where do we learn how to be in touch with and express our feelings?

The "psychology generation" strives to be "in touch" and to "communicate." There was the era of free association, and there was Primal Scream. There are confrontational groups, and there are retreats to help couples share their feelings. There is hypnotherapy and movement therapy and psychotherapy. *Show me how, tell me what to say, tell me what I should do* ---- as if there might be a "DO" prescription for emotions, analogous to the pill prescription for an ulcer or strep throat.

Graduate students of psychotherapy, learning how to treat the emotional problems of prospective patients, listen to tapes made by august professors. They hope to hear sagacious words that will fit emotional quandaries ---- this, as if there were some point-to-point representation, similar to a computer program, that will facilitate a curative emotional experience.

Husbands who find themselves in marital therapy with wives who complain about their lack of feeling, implore, "What do you want me to "DO?" as though "DO" were a passkey to feeling.

Emotions are elusive, and challenging to cope with. The balance of this chapter offers some guidelines.

Guidelines for
Coping with Emotions

Identify the emotion.

To begin to cope with emotions requires first that you identify them. This is not always self-evident, since it is not always clear how to label particular feelings. Fear, anger, guilt, depression ---- all such feelings have their own features that distinguish them. If the feeling is not clear, you might begin by simply noting that "I'm uncomfortable; something isn't right."

Admit the feeling exists.

The next step is to admit to yourself that the feeling exists. Feelings are a natural and normal part of being human.

Accept it.

Acceptance of the feeling is crucial because there is no coping without honesty about what exists. And the most fundamental element of honesty is to be honest with yourself. Sometimes caregivers have trouble accepting their negative emotions because they do not make the distinction between *having* a feeling and *acting* on it. The wish to run away does not mean that one will do it. Being angry at the loved one does not mean that one will be destructive.

Establish distance.

Emotional distress can also be alleviated if you can establish distance from the intensity of the situation. Both physical and emotional distance moderate the feeling of being overwhelmed, hopeless and in constant upheaval. Time away, even a brief walk, can provide the separation necessary to gain objectivity and diffuse emotions.

Emotional distance facilitates a more realistic understanding of what can be expected and what can be accomplished.

Examine it.

Emotions are largely determined by thoughts, attitudes and beliefs. You get angry for a reason; perhaps you think that you've been treated unfairly or you get frustrated because you feel your helpful efforts were rebuffed; or you feel trapped by the thought that the future is hopeless. Your feelings occur because you believe you were wronged. Sometimes you'll find it helpful to examine the reasonableness of your belief. The world, after all, is not always fair, and we must be able to accept this, and go on.

Express it.

Although you may be able to acknowledge negative feelings to yourself, you may be reluctant to express them. Many caregivers are concerned that the expression of feelings will have a negative effect on the relationship. In reality, the basis of a strong relationship is honesty and the expression of feelings. The expression of feelings is an essential part of caregiving.

Nevertheless, it can be very difficult to take the first step in confronting an aged or infirm loved one. As an intermediate step, emotions can be expressed to a friend, a confidant, or a professional. Sometimes intense emotional reactions (e.g., unrelenting depression, immobilizing anxiety) require the assistance of a mental health professional for therapy or medication. These people are able to offer both support and objectivity.

Writing down what one is feeling may help to ventilate and diffuse intense emotions.

Plan something constructive.

Expression should be followed by a plan to do something constructive when the feelings occur. Emotional reactions can interfere with coping by affecting the caregiver's ability to plan. Depression, for example, can lead to problems mobilizing, and can interfere with concentration and motivation. Guilt can interfere with exploring options, such as placement of the loved one. Caregivers must accept that such alternate options are not the same as family care, but that good and genuine care can be given by others. Short-term interventions also require planning so that they can be put into place when feelings of isolation, helplessness, depression, and anger occur. When a plan is formulated in advance, it is more likely that action will be taken when needed.

Strike a balance.

Coping requires striking a balance between being realistic about the illness and maintaining optimism. To cope successfully, you must reach the level of being comfortable that you are doing all that is possible to care for, protect and love the patient while conserving your own resources. This balance is necessary so that you do not slowly deteriorate along with your loved one.

Gain reprieve by living meaningfully.

Adjusting to loss, either of a loved one, or of a part of life as it was previously known, requires that you establish your identity beyond that of being a caregiver. If your sense of self is overly attached to the caregiver role, it will be difficult to accept and work through the loss. To be a caregiver means to confront mortality. To go beyond caregiving is to emotionally reinvest in life, to reach out and relate to others.

We are no different than our loved ones. We all have an amount of time allotted to us between now and the time we die. Reprieve is to live that time in the most honest and meaningful way we can.

8

REAWAKENING

"Awaken: To rouse from a state resembling sleep, as from death ---- To give new life to, to stir up."
(Webster 2nd ed., S.V. "awaken")

Reawaken: To awaken again.

The preceding chapters have looked at the stresses of caregiving and at the associated emotional reactions. Suggestions were offered as to how to cope lest you lose yourself and become too vulnerable. Your feelings told you that to lose yourself in caregiving-created problems: you became depressed, resentful, angry, and lonely. You pushed your feelings away though, because there was no time. Or perhaps you believed it was "wrong" to feel that way.

If you've come this far thinking that the goal was to preserve yourself in order to be a better caregiver, you're missing an important point. You have come to keenly understand the necessity of giving, nurturing, and being sensitive, and you've become an expert in this. Now you must focus your energies on *yourself,* and then go on to find that which nurtures you.

Imagine for a moment that you broke your arm several weeks ago. Now the doctor says, *Your arm was broken. It has mended. Now you must begin to use it again.* But more than just using it, when you awaken and reach your arms over your head, feel how good it is to stretch again.

Being a caregiver meant that, for a while, your life changed: there was less time for you, and other concerns were in the forefront. You tended to another, narrowed your focus, suffered losses, grieved, and perhaps lost sight of the bigger picture. To see the life of a loved one compromised and slip away, however, made it obvious that life is a temporary gift, every aspect of it is time limited. Each of us is born, enters the world, and has a finite end point. Between these points is living and being part of the world.

You have endured disappointment, pain, grief. Now it's time to go on, to *reawaken*, to reconnect in living.

Grief, Loss... and Reawakening

The caregiver grieves the loss of the one who is loved, along with the hopes, dreams and plans connected to that person. To grieve the loss opens up old wounds that were never truly healed. Loss disrupts life as it was, but loss allows us to question the credo of the past. Loss can make us grow, change, and get in touch with our true selves. Loss awakens us to the reality of our impermanence. It can make us question the nature of our existence, our relationship with others, and how we will use the time between now and when we die. When we accept our own mortality and vulnerability, we can accept it in a loved one. It starts inside each of us.

In the Bible, God's first question is, "Adam, where art thou?" God was asking, "Adam, who are you really?" One of Adam's first acts after he bit the apple was to hide and cover his nakedness. Adam felt vulnerable and without worth.

From the Book of Job 1:21: *"Naked, I came from my mother's womb"* ---- without defenses, without a protective shell. Then, like Adam, we learn to cover and hide ourselves, until misfortune strips away our safety and protection. Tragedy and death force us to face our mortality and accept our vulnerability. Stripped of our defenses, our credo and shell, the moment of death is synonymous with reality ---- *"and naked I will depart." (Job: 1:21)*

Loss can mobilize us to attach to life intensely if we become aware that life is temporary. To attach intensely is to feel, think and behave in accordance with our genuine selves. We take the energy which was invested in a loved one and slowly let go of painful memories. We then are left with the good memories and images, and we are ready to reinvest.

To grieve the loss is to begin the process of healing.

The Caring of Others

The paths toward healing vary, but all paths are alike in that they involve sharing with others and not being alone. It is not the advice that others give, or their words of consolation or explanation or mollification or encouragement that heals us; it is their caring ---- whatever they do to show that they care.

February 1993. Nora thought about the day that Sonnie had "happened" to stop by and turned on a late-afternoon talk show. The guests were a panel of women who were recovering alcoholics. A slim, dark-haired, smartly dressed woman spoke about how, for a long time, she had denied her addiction. To concerned friends and relatives, she claimed that she only took an occasional drink to calm her nerves.

Nora listened. After Sonnie left, Nora remembered the small brick building next to the hospital. She picked up the phone and called information. "Can you give me the number for the Alcoholism and Addiction Center of Newport County?"

The Alcoholism and Addiction Center was a local affiliate of Alcoholics Anonymous. At the center they taught healing with the Twelve-Step approach. Nora was comforted by Step Two, which taught that there was a higher power, perhaps God, perhaps the Twelve-Step program itself, that could help. She was glad to find a sponsor at Step Three. Having a sponsor softened the anxiety and loneliness that had first led her to need the numbing effect of alcohol.

March 1993. Step Four. Nora took inventory of herself, her strengths and weaknesses and the vulnerability that made her susceptible to alcohol. Her life had been a series of dependent relationships.

"When I was a child, I learned that if I did what was expected of me, people would love me and take care of me. Later, I needed Glenn so much I would have done anything, so long as he would still be there for me. I thought he liked me that way. I was afraid to be any other way because I thought I would lose the people I needed. I never trusted myself or thought that I could be accepted for my own ideas or decisions."

She could not remember when she had felt really comfortable making a decision. Thrust into the role of caring for Glenn and for herself, she felt as if she were running in a world without shelter. Now she saw that she *had* made decisions and *had* taken care of Glenn. Her fears of being inadequate and incapable were mistaken. She was able to make choices and do what was necessary.

April 1993. The group was discussing the difference between prayer and meditation. Nora remembered her first encounter with meditation. Now she smiled as she envisioned how she must have looked, flying out of the meeting room — now when she was able to look at the fears and the myths.

To pray, they said, was to talk to God "out there." Meditation is to listen to an answer from within one's self. "You can learn to become still, and listen to that quiet, yet powerful voice within you that connects you to your true values in life" (Gorski ,1989).

September 1993. And then she felt changed. Step Twelve is a "spiritual awakening," subtle, yet profound, because thoughts, actions, feelings, attitudes and perceptions change. Step Twelve asks the questions that are inherent in all awakenings. "What is it that you are meant to do with your life? What are your natural talents and beliefs? To what values and purpose do you commit? And finally, how do you reach out to others?"

October 1993. Nora found herself in the small hospital chapel again. Sitting in her regular seat, she recalled when she had been there, perhaps a year before Glenn died. She shuddered, reliving the fear, when fear, like a lost child, was all there was. She remembered how, when Glenn died, she had thought about how easy it would be to sleep in the ground with him.

Now Nora could see light — light streaming through the small, stained glass window, light beaming from two candles on the platform, and light emanating from things alive around her.

Some rows behind her sat a woman, late fortyish, in a flowered dress. Nora took it in, in a glance. The woman's hands were folded in her lap and her shoulders turned inward. Nora noted the fatigue which hung around the woman's body and the way she flicked the side of her eye quickly with a finger. Nora sensed her pain, knowing.

Pardon me as I sit amidst your prayers. Memories now for me, distant from those yearnings and pleas. Tears we may share, though. Mine for the reality of loss, yours of fear and despair. We all must walk from here to there, but no one can tell you how. That is for you to find. Oh, I could tell you about Glenn and what I have learned about going on. But you only know now, this moment, and maybe tomorrow, and that which is your prayer.

In the midst of her calm, Nora felt sympathy for the woman. She got up to leave, detouring to go out the back way, so as to pass the woman. As she did, their eyes met, and Nora stopped and placed her hand on the woman's shoulder. She touched her softly, and whispered, "Take care."

Therapy

Another path toward healing may be with the aid of a trained guide.

September 10, 1992. Fred took a seat in the psychologist's office. He moved uncomfortably in the soft, blue armchair, trying to settle in.

The therapist looked at him casually, but carefully. *Five-foot-ten, medium build, formal in his dark blazer and grey pants.*

Fred placed his feet in parallel alignment as he leaned forward slightly and clasped his hands together in front of his knees.

"Have you ever been to a therapist before?" she asked.

"No. No, never." And to himself, *Never would have believed I would.*

She briefly explained the parameters of therapy: confidentiality, regularly scheduled weekly meetings, initial goal setting. And then she was silent.

He waited. "Well, you know why I'm here."

"Why don't you tell me about it?" she suggested.

And then he talked. Woodenly at first, but then he was surprised at the rush of words and his desire to tell about his life, and how it was when he became the caregiver.

September 24, 1992. Session 3. "You said that at times you found yourself getting angry with Ruth," the therapist said.

"Yes," he acknowledged. "Once she wouldn't put her arm through her sleeve. Maybe she couldn't, but I didn't think of that then. I was just getting so frustrated and mad. Mad trying to put her arm through her sleeve. I thought, 'She's making it tough.' Finally I shook her. I got so mad I just shook her. I wanted to yell, but she was so afraid. I felt so bad, I just sat down, still. I couldn't move. I knew I did wrong. I felt bad, but I still got mad times after that. I got so I was afraid I would really hurt her."

October 8, 1992. Session 5. "After the first time I hurt Ruth I was so upset, but I would still get angry and sometimes be rough with her again. I felt guilty. I couldn't believe what I had done, even when it was more than once. It was like there was someone else. Someone I would never have believed existed. I was not in control.

"At night, I couldn't sleep. I would ask God, 'How can this happen? How could I have done it again?' I would ask for help and forgiveness, for pardon."

There are no pardons. There are only reprieves.

November 12, 1992. Session 10. "I love golf." Fred was talking to the therapist. "When I get on the golf course, I forget everything. It's my escape.

"Three mornings a week, they would pick her up and take her to day care and I could get things done. Sometimes get in a round of golf. Before Ruth became really sick, those mornings saved me.

"One day, I was getting her dressed, putting her shoes on. She kept moving her foot so that I couldn't get the angle. I think she liked to give me a hard time when I was dressing her. We were running late already, and I was worried that we'd miss the pickup bus. I guess I could have driven her myself, but I didn't think of it. I got angry. I was so frustrated. I wanted to get out to play some golf. I took her foot and jammed it into the shoe. She jerked her foot back. I was angry at her because, again, she had forced me to be rough. She stepped down on the foot and kind of jumped. I was afraid they'd notice at the day care. I kept her home and put ice on her ankle. I felt trapped and miserable."

December 10, 1992. Session 13. "How have you been doing?" Dr. Golden asked.

Fred sat down, feeling looser than usual. "My granddaughter told me a joke. You want to hear it?"

Dr. Golden nodded ambivalently.

"Knock, knock."

Dr. Golden waited four seconds. "O.K. Who's there?"

"Sarah."

"Sarah, who?"

"Sarah doctor in the house?"

After minimal response, Fred continued. "Maybe you'll like the one about Mr. Gluck who went to his therapist complaining about a problem with short-term memory."

Dr. Golden listened.

"'I don't seem to have any,' said Gluck. 'How long have your had the problem?' asked the therapist. Gluck looked at the therapist, puzzled. 'What problem?'"

Now Dr. Golden chuckled and Fred continued. "I've been feeling better about things. When I saw Ruth today she smiled and looked happy. They take good care of her at the nursing home. I thought she recognized me when I walked in. Maybe not. Maybe she was just in a good mood and was smiling an old Ruthie smile.

"Today I realized I couldn't do all she needed any more. She needs a lot of care."

Faith as Healer

Faith is another road to healing. Faith allows us to look at things in the light and to release our fears from the shadows, where they are magnified.

"When we pray to God we speak the words in our heart, and thus gain access to our inner selves. A prayer is a plumbline, dropped to the center of the soul, a line to disclose our inner depths." (Wolpe, 1992)

In healing, we turn to God or a greater power not for answers or reward, but rather for a sense that we are not alone. When we reach inside through prayer, meditation or self-exploration, we draw on our own strength and courage. We accept that life is not perfect or free of pain, and that the world is not always logical or orderly. But reawakening to life is our chance to find peace, pleasure, and fulfillment. In reconnecting to life, we realize that we are part of something more grand and more enduring than ourselves.

As a caregiver you have done more than struggle; you have learned. You are sensitized to time. Hold it in your palm and take it for yourself. You are sensitized to nurturing. Invest in caring for yourself. You are sensitized to loss. Embrace the things that matter to you. Reawaken to the simple things ---- the feeling of the sun on your face and the breeze on your body, the sound of a bird, the rhythm of a song. Rediscover someone from the past. Love something new. Let your mind wander free to find a new dream ---- one you can have; it will come to you. Take the first small, real step toward it, then the next.

In *War and Peace*, Tolstoy's central character, Pierre, seeks to understand the individual's place and meaning in life. Pierre speaks to his friend, the disillusioned Prince Andre, of his discovery.

> *"'If there is a God and future life, there is truth and good, and man's highest happiness consists in striving to attain them. We must live, we must love, and we must believe that we live not only today on this scrap of earth, but have lived and shall live forever, there, in the Whole,' said Pierre, and he pointed to the sky."* (Tolstoy, 1942)

On Pierre's return to Moscow, at the end of the Napoleonic War, he states:

> *"Life is everything. Life is God. To love life is to love God. Harder, and more blessed than all else is to love this life in one's sufferings, in innocent sufferings."* (Tolstoy, 1942)

If loss causes us to look deep inside and discover our genuine selves, if it makes us aware of our resources and our ability to love and care, if it makes us reattach intensely to the world around us, then our loved one becomes a testimony to life, rather than a source of despair. *And this is the caregiver's reprieve.*

EPILOGUE

Clear April morning. Spring breezes nudging out winter.

Brian was getting ready for his first day working part time at Taggart's. Becca noticed the clothes he had chosen. He looked fine. She held back when he picked up a light jacket that might not insulate him from the morning crispness.

"I'm off! See you later." He stepped out quickly without hesitation, despite the awkwardness of his gait, like the Brian of old, and was out the door.

Becca felt a mixture of tension and joy as she watched him go off in the direction of the bus stop to take the short walk they had rehearsed many times. Now she resisted her desire to walk with him some of the way on this first day he would be going by himself. She was reassured knowing that the bus would let him off right in front of Taggart's.

Brian reached the bus stop. Soon, over the crest of the hill, he saw the top of the bus. He felt in his pocket, and his fingers circled the rims of the two quarters.

Becca opened the back door to the first scent of spring air and the chirping of a sparrow on the railing of the porch. It reminded her of a brown bird they had found one frigid January, stuck to the ice on the driveway. The surface of the roads and walkways had been thick with ice and non-navigable. The ice refused to thaw and had brought everything to a halt, including the brown bird whose wing had become fused to the ice in the driveway. They had covered the bird with a cloth and then thawed the ice with warm water, thus freeing the bird which flew away in a flourish.

Now Becca thought, There are always birds around that side of the house. But this brown, chirping harbinger of spring really looked like the one that they had set free!

POSTSCRIPT 1997

Becca

I know that our life is forever changed by the continued need to look after Brian, but the important thing for me is that I have learned to accept things and people the way they are ---- to appreciate people's weaknesses as well as their strengths and to focus on the simple moments of happiness in life.

Nora

It's been nine years since Glenn was first diagnosed. I have changed. I discovered that I have faith in myself, I can trust my instincts, and I believe in my basic self worth. I understand better who I am and what I'm doing with my life, and that is what really matters.

Fred

I remember when Ruth first became ill. I thought I could change things back if only I had a plan and took good care of her. Now I realize that you can't always be in control. What's more, it's good to let go sometimes and lighten up. I feel better.

Woody

I never thought about it in the early years when I was taking care of Mam, but now I know that an important part of life is giving and taking. The best thing I do for Mam is simply to be there, to care for her. Sometimes it feels like you give a lot more than you get, so be good to yourself, too!

APPENDICES

The following appendices may provide useful information for you in the course of your caregiving.

Many of the conditions which render a loved one seriously impaired involve the brain and central nervous system. A description of their anatomy and functioning are given in Appendix A.

Numerous medical conditions require extensive caregiving. A description of some of these, while not exhaustive, is found in Appendix B.

In the course of a loved one's illness, diagnostic procedures may be necessary in order to identify and evaluate the condition. Some of these are described in Appendix C.

The terms described in Appendices B and C are found in the *American Medical Association Encyclopedia of Medicine*, a good general reference that is easy to read and inclusive.

Appendix D suggests resources, including agencies, organizations, and literature, which can provide support and information.

APPENDIX A

THE BRAIN IS A WONDROUS ORGAN

One of the more difficult adjustments for caregivers is associated with the loved one's cognitive and personality changes. To help the reader understand these changes, information about the neurological basis of behavior is provided.

From its position at the top of the body, the brain controls all functions beneath it. Possessing what has been speculated to be billions of nerve cells, with an estimated potential for trillions of connections, the brain is a wondrous organ.

As processing center, the brain is both more intricate and more numerous in its connections than anything that has ever been constructed, including the most sophisticated super-computer. Yet, unlike a computer, the brain is alive, has self determination, and is not limited by preprogramming. Seemingly endless in the bits of information it can generate, it is also the most complex natural phenomenon known.

The intricate structure of the *homo sapiens* brain is determined by genetic codes which result in uniformity of the ridges, grooves, areas and pathways of the human brain. Within every brain, however, is an original assemblage of thoughts, memories and emotions.

The way you pace your words, your recollection of your first day at school, your sense of rhythm and pitch, whether you smile or shake hands when you meet someone new, whether you hold on tightly or barely touch, the memory of your father's face and endless perceptions, choices, feelings and memories are stored in the cells and pathways of each brain in a unique pattern.

The brain and the spinal cord comprise the central nervous system (CNS). The CNS takes in messages from the outside world via the sense organs (eyes, ears, nose and skin). The CNS then transmits messages from the brain back to the organs and muscles for action.

Both the brain and the spinal cord are protected by bones (the skull and vertebrae, respectively), by membranes, and by a cushioning fluid called cerebrospinal fluid. This fluid is also found in the ventricles of the brain.

The basic anatomical unit of the central nervous system is the neuron, or nerve cell. Every nerve cell has a cell body, one long projection (the *axon*), and many short projections (called *dendrites.)* Axons band together to form tracts of "white matter," which connect parts of the brain and spinal cord. Thus axons and dentrites also allow for a multiplicity of connections between nerve cells over which "messages" travel within the brain. These multiple connections account for the vast storage of information in the brain.

The transmission of a message from one cell to another has been compared to an electrical circuit. The association between nerve cells involves electrical and chemical reactions and constitutes the nerve impulse. The impulse travels down the length of the axon to the dendrite of an adjacent cell. At the end of the axon, the neuron releases a chemical called a *neurotransmitter.* This chemical moves across the space between cells and sets off the reaction in the next cell.

Structurally, the brain is a three-and-a-half-pound mass of soft, sponge-like tissue. It consists of three distinct, but interconnected, sections ---- the *cerebral cortex,* the *cerebellum* and the *brain stem.* The brain stem and midbrain are responsible for the automatic control of vital functions (including respiration, heart beat, blood pressure, body temperature, hunger, thirst and sleep).

This section, then, maintains homeostasis, or a state of equilibrium, in the body.

The cerebellum, which lies beneath and to the rear of the cortex, is involved in coordination and balance.

Higher functions, such as decision making, thinking and perception are found at the level of the cerebral cortex. At this level the brain takes in information, decides how to respond, and then implements the response.

The surface of the cerebral cortex contains a large number of grooves which expand the surface area and thus increase the amount of information which can be stored. The cerebral cortex is divided into two halves, called hemispheres, which generally control the opposite side of the body. The hemispheres are connected by nerve pathways which coordinate the activity of both sides of the brain. Typically, one hemisphere is considered to be dominant and slightly more developed than the other. This is usually the left hemisphere. It contains the speech centers which are responsible for the reception and expression of language, and it determines hand preference.

Research on the hemispheres has established the existence of functions intrinsic to each. Right hemisphere functions include spatial orientation and awareness, recognizing shapes, sense of music and rhythm, appreciation of humor and emotion, sense of time, and discrimination of colors. The left hemisphere controls the reception and expression of language, including the ability to read, write and speak. It is, therefore, responsible for the analysis and processing of verbal information in all modalities.

Within each hemisphere, the brain is further subdivided into *lobes*. The *frontal lobe*, so named because of its location, is the center for the integration of information. It is the locus for attention and for the planning, initiation, and evaluation of voluntary behavior. It is also responsible for the inhibition of inappropriate behavior. A deep groove separates the frontal lobe from the *parietal lobe*. In front of the groove is the *motor cortex*, which controls voluntary movement in the body. Behind the groove, in the parietal lobe, is the *sensory cortex*, which receives sensations of touch, pressure, temperature, pain and position. The parietal lobes integrate sensation and movement and are responsible for visual/spatial orientation, the recognition of faces and of familiar objects.

The processing of auditory information occurs in the *temporal lobe*, which is located in the vicinity of the ear. The left temporal lobe typically contains the speech centers which decode, analyze and integrate language. The right temporal lobe is involved in decoding of visual information and the appreciation of music. The temporal lobes are also a location for memory functions.

At the back of the brain is the *occipital lobe*. The cortex of the occipital lobe codes, integrates and synthesizes visual information.

Within each lobe, areas are further designated as primary, secondary and tertiary. Primary areas receive sensations from the body and the outside world. The secondary areas then organize the information and give it meaning. Finally, the tertiary areas take the pieces of information from the secondary areas and integrate them with information from other secondary areas, thus giving meaning to more complex, higher, cognitive functions.

Modern neuropsychologists adopt a view of the brain as composed of "functional systems." Anatomically, these systems are composed of cortical and subcortical areas which work in concert to produce a behavior or function. Damage to any area of the system can disrupt many functions and, as a corollary, damage to a specific part of the system results in specific signs and symptoms. The brain, though, has a certain amount of "plasticity" or ability to reorganize. The implication of this is that, after injury, the brain can be retrained to find an alternate route to perform the function.

APPENDIX B

THE BRAIN WHEN THINGS GO WRONG

Several physical conditions result in dementia, the progressive decline of intellectual functioning. Symptoms of dementia include memory loss, confusion, personality changes, and impairment of cognitive functions including judgment, reasoning, abstract thinking, spatial orientation and language uses.

Underlying causes of dementia include damage to brain tissue, vascular disease, structural problems, infections, degenerative diseases of the brain, metabolic disease and psychiatric disorders.

Cerebral Vascular Disease

Stroke

A stroke, or *cerebro-vascular accident* (CVA), is a disease involving the arterial circulation of the brain. The onset of stroke is sudden. It occurs when a blood vessel in the brain bursts, causing a hemorrhage, or when a blood vessel becomes clogged with a clot (thrombus). Typically, a stroke occurs in an artery which has been damaged by arteriosclerosis (the progressive buildup of fatty deposits on its walls). The narrowed artery, which is already delivering a restricted blood supply to the brain, is vulnerable to the closing effect of a thrombus.

Factors which predispose an individual to stroke are elevated cholesterol and blood lipid levels, high blood pressure, and diabetes.

In a CVA, the blockage or the hemorrhage of blood vessels in the brain interrupts the flow of oxygen to the brain and can result in tissue death. The effects of stroke may be permanent or temporary. Typically, the more widespread the deficits, the poorer the prognosis.

The most common effects of stroke are impairment in motor, sensory and speech functions. Loss of motor and sensory functions are typically manifested on the opposite side of the body from the hemisphere in which the stroke occurred. In addition to the loss of control of physical functions, stroke patients may show signs of dementia, including memory lapses, impaired judgement, and intellectual decline. Emotional changes, including periods of depression and intermittent loss of emotional control, may also be evident.

Recovery after stroke depends on how quickly the supply of blood is returned to the affected area and how well other areas of the brain take over functions of the affected area.

TIA

TIA, or *transient ischemic attack*, is another type of cerebro-vascular disease. A TIA is a brief interruption in the blood supply to the brain. This may be followed by a momentary, barely noticeable, loss of ability to function. The affects of TIA, however, build up over time, as the number of incidents increase. Individuals with TIAs that go untreated are likely candidates for a stroke at a later date.

Head Injury

Brain damage occurs very frequently as a result of head injury. Because the brain is extremely sensitive to trauma, even a mild head injury can have long term consequences. In head injury, damage occurs when the head snaps and pushes the brain against the skull. Blood vessels are torn, and brain tissue swells and is compressed against the skull. Brain tissues can be destroyed by direct impact or by the bleeding associated with the injury. Severe head injury is almost always accompanied by a period of unconsciousness, the duration of which generally reflects the severity of the underlying brain damage. Frequently, there is amnesia for the events immediately preceding the incident (retrograde amnesia) and for a period of time after consciousness is regained (anterograde amnesia).

Brain injury can be either focal or diffuse. If it is focal, damage occurs at the point of impact, and deficits are specific to the location of the damage. Neurological signs of focal damage include impairments in motor skills, sensation, coordination, or whatever function is associated with the area damaged. Diffuse injury, in which there is widespread damage, is due to the shearing of the axons in the white matter. Diffuse brain injury is usually accompanied by brain swelling and edema, and typically disturbs the whole brain. Psychological problems which accompany head injury include difficulties with memory, concentration, impulsiveness, irritability and emotional problems.

Traumatic injury may also occur in the brain stem, causing disturbances in respiration, circulation, and other vital functions. Observed outcomes of brain stem injury include the slowing of heart rate, irregular breathing, changes in blood pressure and metabolic changes.

The outcome of head injury depends on the severity and nature of the injury, length of unconsciousness, age of the patient, and medical interventions.

There are three basic types of brain injury: *lacerations, contusions* and *concussions*.

Laceration

A laceration occurs when the brain has been penetrated. The ensuing damage is restricted to the affected focal area. Lacerations can cause permanent damage. The resulting scar tissue in the brain has the potential to become a point of irritation and, consequently, a locus for seizure activity.

Concussion

A concussion is the result of a blow to the head and is usually followed by a brief loss of consciousness. This can have diverse effects on mental functioning.

Contusion

A contusion is a more serious injury. The damage and bleeding associated with contusion occur both locally and to the opposite hemisphere. This is due to the thrusting of the brain against the opposite side of the skull. The latter produces a syndrome called "contrecoup," which results from the tearing of blood vessels between the brain and surrounding membranes.

With time, as brain swelling diminishes and diffuse effects abate, the results of head injury are associated with the particular area of damage. Permanent deficits then are more specific and may include loss of sensory and motor function, impaired speech and language skills, residual memory deficits which persist after the amnesias clear, slowed reaction time, visual/perceptual deficits, and post-traumatic psychiatric disorders. Examples of the latter are headache, dizziness, irritability, insomnia, confusional states and anxiety.

Increased Intracranial Pressure

Injury to the brain may lead to a buildup of fluids, which increases the pressure inside the skull. This occurs when blood vessels rupture and blood accumulates. The accumulation of blood is called a *hematoma* and can occur between the membranes of the brain or within the brain itself.

Pressure can also build up because of an accumulation of cerebrospinal fluid. Since the skull is rigid, there is no room to relieve the pressure. Surgical intervention to relieve the pressure can prevent further tissue damage.

Tumor

A brain tumor is an expanding mass that can begin either in the brain or in some other part of the body. Tumor cells travel to the brain via the blood stream. The symptoms manifested are generally due to compression of the surrounding tissue. Brain tumors follow a progressive course characterized by either an intensification of a symptom or an increase in the number of symptoms. The rate of growth of the tumor may be slow or rapid, varying from weeks to years. Slow-growing tumors may not produce symptoms for a long time. The effects of tumors are generally related to the location and the size of the tumor.

Tumors are divided into two categories, non-infiltrative and infiltrative. The effects of non-infiltrative tumors are due to their growth and eventual compression of brain tissue to the point where a function is interrupted. Infiltrative tumors are more diffuse in their effects. Tumors of the glial, or supportive, cells of the brain, for example, grow quite rapidly, quickly destroying brain tissue and resulting in a general decline of intellectual functions.

Tumors are graded according to their rate of growth or malignancy. A grade 1 tumor is slow growing, while a grade 4 tumor, for example, a glioblastoma, quickly produces symptoms.

Metastatic tumors originate in other parts of the body, such as the lungs or breast, and can metastasize to several areas of the brain. The early picture can begin with a variety of symptoms. However, as the disease progresses, there is widespread loss of function.

Dementia

Dementia is a term used to describe a marked deterioration of mental abilities affecting many areas of the brain. In progressive dementias, the loss of cognitive abilities continues to the point at which the individual is totally unable to handle self-care.

Early signs of dementia include gradual loss of memory, disturbance in speech, and problems with spatial orientation. These early losses can be picked up on formal psychological testing before they become apparent in behavioral changes observed at home or in the workplace.

As the dementia progresses, judgment and reasoning become impaired. The individual then is unable to process new information or adjust to change. Personality changes are common. They may be manifested as an exaggeration of previous traits or in the appearance of a trait not observed in the pre-existing personality. Individuals suffering from dementia often become listless, dependent, fearful, demanding and irritable.

In the early stages of dementia, problems with verbal expression increase and self-help skills are gradually lost.

Eventually, impaired motor functioning renders the individual bedridden, and nursing care becomes necessary.

Alzheimer's Disease

Alzheimer's disease is perhaps the most prevalent example of a progressive, irreversible dementia. Characteristic changes in brain tissue in Alzheimer's patients include the formation of abnormal deposits called plaques and the presence of tangled bundles of nerve fibers. Recent research on Alzheimer's has discovered neurochemical and protein abnormalities, as well as deficiencies of neurotransmitters in the brain. Degeneration and loss of brain cells have been found in several brain areas, namely those involved in short-term memory and various other cognitive functions.

The onset of Alzheimer's is insidious and, as with other dementias, early signs may first be attributed to forgetfulness, laziness or depression. The course of the disease and the rate of decline vary. The illness can progress for a period of five to twenty years before total incapacitation and death ensue.

Over time, cognitive losses affect thinking, judgement, reasoning, memory and language expression. As with other dementias, there are notable personality and motor changes, the latter progressing to the point where the patient is totally dependent, bedridden, and susceptible to serious infection.

Thus far there is no treatment that stops the progression of Alzheimer's. Medications can be prescribed however, to improve sleep and reduce emotional volatility, depression, and wandering.

Multi-Infarct Dementia

Cognitive impairment associated with multi-infarct dementia is the result of a series of small strokes over time. The accompanying reduced blood flow to parts of the brain causes oxygen deprivation and subsequent tissue death. The changes that result from one episode may be negligible. With additional incidents, however, the changes are cumulative, eventually affecting mental functions and interfering with memory.

The clinical picture that emerges may be indistinguishable from that of Alzheimer's disease; in fact, multi-infarct dementia, at times, is found in combination with Alzheimer's.

Typically, symptoms of multi-infarct dementia include problems with memory, coordination and speech. Unlike the steady, progressive deterioration found in Alzheimer's, multi-infarct dementia seems to advance in a step-wise manner. The patient appears worse after an incident, and then symptoms level off until another incident.

Predisposing factors to multi-infarct dementia include high blood pressure, diabetes, cigarette smoking, high cholesterol and impaired cardiac functioning.

While multi-infarct dementia is progressive, it may respond to treatment with medications which reduce the incidence of further strokes. Research has indicated that low doses of aspirin may be effective in retarding the progress of the disease by reducing the probability of new strokes.

AIDS-Related Dementia

AIDS, or Acquired Immune Deficiency Syndrome, is caused by a virus ---- the Human Immunodeficiency Virus (HIV) ---- which attacks the immune system. The weakened immune system makes the individual susceptible to other diseases, which become the actual cause of death.

AIDS-related dementia is thought to have two underlying mechanisms. One, it is speculated that the AIDS virus actually attacks the brain cells; and two, impairment of the immune system makes the brain susceptible to infection and subsequent encephalitis.

AIDS-related dementia is slow developing and may evolve over a period of five to ten years. Eventually, in the later stages of the disease, cognitive functions become impaired.

Non-dementia Producing Disorders of the Central Nervous System

Unlike many of the already noted impairments of the Central Nervous System, there are a number of pathological conditions of the CNS which leave cognitive functioning relatively unimpaired.

Several of these, such as cerebral palsy, multiple sclerosis and Parkinson's Disease, primarily affect motor functioning.

Multiple Sclerosis

Multiple sclerosis is a chronic and, at times, progressive disease of the nervous system which can be debilitating but not cognitively impairing. Symptoms are primarily physical. The disease can be precipitated by a genetic or postnatal event such as trauma or infection.

MS is a disease which affects the axons, or tracts, of the CNS. The axons are insulated by a white sheath called myelin, which facilitates the conduction of the nerve impulse from nerve fiber to nerve fiber. In MS, areas of the myelin sheath become inflamed, destroyed and subsequently replaced by scar tissue. The presence of the scar (sclerosis) interferes with the conduction of the nerve impulse, thus making it difficult to execute and control movement.

The diagnosis of MS is made with the help of CAT Scans, MRI, evoked potential testing, and spinal taps. While these tests locate areas of lesion, it frequently takes multiple attacks, over time, to establish the diagnosis of MS.

Symptoms of MS are predominantly motor, including problems with balance and coordination, general weakness and speech disorders. Fatigue and lack of energy are especially problematic and appear to be aggravated by hot and humid weather. Sensory symptoms such as numbness, pins and needles, and visual problems may also be present.

MS progresses at a different rate from person to person. In its most benign course, after a few initial attacks there is little disability. There are also cases in which repeated attacks cause some disability but are followed by periods of remission which may last for some time. Finally there is a course in which there is steady, albeit slow, progression of the disease without remission.

While new treatments and drugs for MS are being developed, there is still no cure.

Parkinson's Disease

Parkinson's Disease is a neurological condition involving the motor cortex of the brain and, therefore, predominantly causing disturbances in movement. The symptoms of Parkinson's include uncontrolled tremors, stiffness, slowness of movement, and change in facial expression. Deterioration in Parkinson's occurs in stages. Initially this is evidenced by a mild tremor of a limb at rest.

As the disease progresses, overall movement is slowed and posture is stooped. Later in the disease, balance problems are notable, and there is a tendency to fall. Finally, motor ability is significantly impaired. Performance on tests of cognitive ability are initially mildly compromised, however later in the disease, there is a general impairment of intellectual functions.

Patients with Parkinson's are found to have reduced amounts of the neurotransmitter Dopamine in the brain. L-Dopa, a drug which raises Dopamine levels in the brain, tends to help with the sensory/motor deficits and slows down the progress of the disease.

Hydrocephalus

Increased pressure from cerebro-spinal fluid in the ventricles of the brain produces a condition known as hydrocephalus. Hydrocephalus is classified as either primary or secondary. In primary, or normal pressure hydrocephalus, no underlying disease or structural basis is identified, although the ventricles appear to be quite enlarged. Secondary hydrocephalus results from, or is secondary to, some other condition of the brain ---- such as head injury, infection, structural blockage, or hemorrhage ---- in which the flow of cerebrospinal fluid is obstructed. The characteristic triad of symptoms in hydrocephalus is intellectual deterioration (primarily in the form of memory deficits), shuffling gait and incontinence. Symptoms intensify as the ventricles continue to expand and exert pressure on surrounding brain tissue.

Some success in ameliorating this condition has been obtained with a shunt operation in which a tube is inserted in the ventricular system of the brain, thus draining off excess cerebrospinal fluid and relieving the pressure.

APPENDIX C

LOOKING INSIDE

The diagnosis and evaluation of brain disease is made by using a variety of laboratory tests. In recent years these procedures have become quite sophisticated and provide invaluable information about the disease process.

Electroencephalogram (EEG)

An EEG is a recording of the electrical activity of the brain. It is a painless procedure whereby readings are obtained through electrodes which are attached to the scalp. The EEG measures patterns of brain waves. Various brain waves or rhythms are associated with particular states of the brain, such as sleep and wake, as well as stages of alertness and concentration.

The EEG is helpful in locating areas of stroke, epilepsy and tumor damage, since it can pick up the abnormal electrical activity associated with these conditions.

Lumbar Puncture (Spinal Tap)

This procedure, done under local anesthesia, is one in which cerebrospinal fluids are extracted from the spinal cord. The fluid is then analyzed to determine whether there is an infection in the central nervous system.

Computerized Axial Tomography (CAT) Scan

The CAT Scan is a sophisticated X-ray. It produces a series of images of the brain from many angles. It is capable of producing thousands of cross-sections of the brain in seconds. These cross-sections are computer analyzed by comparing the relative density of brain tissue. The comparison is then used to distinguish healthy from unhealthy tissue.

CAT Scans are capable of picking up details of the soft tissue of the brain, thus delineating the exact location of damage. It is, therefore, used to find evidence of stroke, atrophy, hemorrhage, tumor and multi-infarct dementia and to identify changes in the size of the ventricles and in the flow of cerebrospinal fluid.

The CAT Scan is far superior to conventional X-rays in the amount of detail obtained, while not necessitating any more exposure to radioactivity than conventional X-rays.

Magnetic Resonance Imaging (MRI)

MRI is a type of scanning device that uses electromagnetic waves to produce a measurable picture of the hydrogen atoms in the scanned area of the body (e.g., the brain). The human body is about 60% water, and there are two hydrogen atoms in every molecule of water. No x-rays are involved and no "radiation" ---- in the conventional sense of that term ---- is sent through the tissues. Information from the scan is used to compose a computerized image yielding precise anatomical detail ---- even of soft tissue. Because diseased cells react differently to the magnetic resonance, healthy tissue can be distinguished from diseased tissue. The MRI is especially useful for picking up lesions in the brain, as well as for finding internal bleeding and for observing blood flow.

Positron Tomography (PET) Scan

An exciting new imaging tool is the PET Scan. Unlike CAT Scan and MRI, which indicate anatomical structure, the PET Scan actually gives a picture of the brain at work. The PET Scan is sensitive to metabolic activity of the brain and thus indicates how parts of the brain are functioning. The images obtained by a PET

Scan are based on the brain's use of glucose for metabolism. The more active the brain is, the more glucose it uses.

PET Scan uses radioactively tagged glucose, which is injected into the bloodstream. The glucose travels to the brain and is then taken up by active cells. A computer picture is made of how the brain is metabolizing this source of energy. This shows which parts of the brain are working during any given mental activity or condition.

PET Scan is particularly useful in assessing a disease process. By demonstrating which parts of the brain are not working well, it can indicate the presence of brain disease. In some instances PET Scans have been able to indicate the extent of tissue damage with more accuracy than CAT Scan.

The PET Scan is being used in research to identify areas of the brain that are associated with particular mental functions and emotional states. It is also being used to discover the location of thoughts and memories. Research also suggests that the PET Scan is a promising diagnostic tool for differentiating various psychological problems.

APPENDIX D

RESOURCES

Associations

Alzheimer's Association. 919 N. Michigan Ave., Suite 100, Chicago, Illinois 60611-1676. 1-800-272-3900.

American Cancer Society. 1599 Clifton Road, NE. Atlanta, Georgia 30329-4251. 1-800-ACS-2345.

American Parkinson's Disease Association, Inc. 1250 Hylan Boulevard, Suite 4B, Staten Island, New York 10305-1946. 1-800-223-2732.

Family Caregiver Alliance. 425 Bush Street, Ste. 500, San Francisco, California 94108. 415-434-3388.

Multiple Sclerosis Association of America. 706 Haddenfield Road, Cherry Hill, New Jersey 08002. 1-800-833-4672.

National Brain Tumor Foundation. 785 Market Street. Suite 1600, San Francisco, California 84103. 1-800-934-CURE.

National Cancer Institute. 9000 Rockville Pike, 30 Center Drive - MSC 22580, Bethesda, Maryland 20892-2580. 1-800-422-6237.

National Family Caregivers Association. 9621 E. Bexhill Dr., Kensington, Maryland 20895. 1-800-535-3198.

Literature

Burger, Sarah Green, et al. & The National Citizens' Coalition for Nursing Home Reform. *Nuring Homes: Getting Good Care There.* Impact Publishers, Inc., San Luis Obispo, California, 1996.

Greutzner, Howard. *Alzheimer's: A Caregiver's Guide and Source Book.* John Wiley and Son. New York. 1992.

Karr, Katherine. *Taking Time for Me.* Prometheus Books. Buffalo, New York. 1992.

Smith, Kerri S. *Caring for Your Aging Parents: A Sourcebook of Timesaving Techniques and Tips.* Impact Publishers, Inc., San Luis Obispo, California, 1994.

Walker, Susan. *Keeping Active: A Caregiver's Guide to Activities with the Elderly.* Impact Publishers, Inc., San Luis Obispo, California. 1994.

BIBLIOGRAPHY

Arieti, Silvana, ed. 1966. *American Handbook of Psychiatry*. New York: Basic Books.

AARP. 1985. *Helping an Aged Loved One*. Illinois: Scott, Foresman and Co.

Beattie, Melody. 1990. *Codependents' Guide to the Twelve Steps*. New York: Prentice Hall.

Benson, Herbert, M.D. 1975. *The Relaxation Response*. New York: Avon.

Berhein, Kayla, Beale, Caroline T., Lewine, Richard, R.J. 1982. *The Caring Family: Living with Chronic Mental Illness*. New York: Random House.

Bloomfield, Harold H., M.D., Cain, Michael Peter, & Jaffee, Dennis T. 1975. *Discovering Inner Energy and Overcoming Stress*. New York: Delacorte Press.

Caplan, Bruce. 1987. *Rehabilitation Desk Reference*. Rockville, Maryland: Aspen Publications.

Clayman, Charles, M.D., Medical Editor. 1989. *The American Medical Association Encyclopedia of Medicine*. New York: Random House.

Cohen, Donna, Ph.D., & Eisdorfer, Carl, Ph.D., M.D. 1986. *The Loss of the Self*. New York: W.W. Norton and Company.

Cristall, Barbara. 1992. *Coping When a Parent Has Multiple Sclerosis*. New York: Rosen Publishing Group.

Doernberg, Myra. 1986. *Stolen Mind: The Slow Disappearance of Ray Doernberg.* Chapel Hill: Algonquin Books.

Gorski, Terence T. 1989. *Understanding the Twelve Steps.* New York: Prentice Hall.

Griffin, Moria. 1989. *Going the Distance.* New York: E.P. Dutton.

Gruetzner, Howard. 1992. *Alzheimer's: A Caregiver's Guide and Sourcebook.* New York: John Wiley & Sons.

Heston, Leonard C., M.D., & White, June A. 1983. *Dementia, a Practical Guide to Alzheimer's Disease and Related Illnesses.* New York: W.H. Freeman and Co.

Jung, Carl G. 1923. *Psychological Types.* New York: Harcourt, Brace, and Co.

Karr, Katherine. 1992. *Taking Time for Me.* New York: Prometheus Books.

Kushner, Harold. 1983. *When Bad Things Happen to Good People.* New York: Avon Books.

Lavin, John H. 1985. *Stroke —— from Crisis to Victory: A Family Guide.* New York: Franklin Watts.

Lezak, Muriel D. 1988. Brain Damage is a Family Affair. *Journal of Clinical and Experimental Neuropsychology.* 10: 111-123.

Lezak, Muriel D. 1978. Life with the characterologically altered brain injured patient. *Journal of Clinical Psychiatry.* 39: 592-598.

Mace, Nancy L., M.A., & Rabins, Peter M., M.D., M.P.H. 1981. *The 36-Hour Day.* New York: Johns Hopkins University Press.

Maharishi Mahesh Yogi 1970-1973. Videotaped residence course lecture. Series, Tapes available through International Film and Tape Library.

Monroe, Ruth. 1955. *Schools of Psychoanalytic Thought.* New York: Holt, Rinehart, and Winston.

Moses, Ken, Ph.D. 1992. *Shattered Dreams and Growth: A Workshop on Helping and Being Helped*. Evanston, Illinois: Resource Network.

Sanders, Catherine M., Ph.D. 1989. *Grief: The Mourning After. Dealing with Adult Bereavement*. New York: John Wiley and Sons.

Seymour, Claire. 1983. *Precipice: Learning to Live with Alzheimer's Disease*. New York: Vantage Press.

Sisk, Ginny. 1992. *This Too Shall Pass: Being a Caregiver for the Elderly*. Nashville: Broadman Press.

Susik, Helen. 1995. *Hiring Home Caregivers*. San Luis Obispo, California: Impact Publishers, Inc.

Tolstoy, Leo. 1942. *War and Peace*. New York: Simon and Schuster.

Webster, Barbara D. 1989. *All of a Piece: A Life with Multiple Sclerosis*. Baltimore: Johns Hopkins University Press.

Wolman, Benjamin B., ed. 1955. *Handbook of Clinical Psychology*. New York: McGraw Hill.

Wolpe, David 1992. *In Speech and in Silence*. New York: Henry Holt.

INDEX